ABC of
# HIV and AIDS

**Sixth Edition**

# ABC series

An outstanding collection of resources – written by specialists for non-specialists

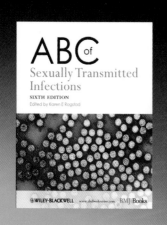

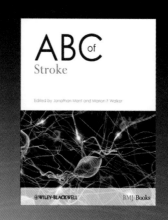

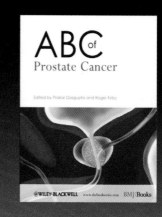

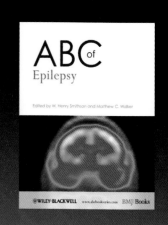

The *ABC* series contains a wealth of indispensable resources for GPs, GP registrars, junior doctors, doctors in training and all those in primary care

▶ **Now fully revised and updated**
▶ **Highly illustrated, informative and a practical source of knowledge**
▶ **An easy-to-use resource, covering the symptoms, investigations, treatment and management of conditions presenting in day-to-day practice and patient support**
▶ **Full colour photographs and illustrations aid diagnosis and patient understanding of a condition**

For more information on all books in the *ABC* series, including links to further information, references and links to the latest official guidelines, please visit:

www.abcbookseries.com

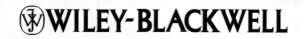

BMJ|Books

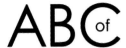

# ABC of

# HIV and AIDS

## Sixth Edition

EDITED BY

### Michael W. Adler

Emeritus Professor of Genitourinary Medicine/Sexually Transmitted Diseases
University College London Medical School
London, UK

### Simon G. Edwards

Consultant GU/HIV Physician
Camden Provider Services
Mortimer Market Centre
London, UK

### Robert F. Miller

Professor, Reader in Clinical Infection and Honorary Consultant Physician
University College London Medical School
London, UK

### Gulshan Sethi

Consultant Physician in Sexual Health and HIV
Guy's and St Thomas' NHS Foundation Trust
London, UK

### Ian G. Williams

Senior Lecturer and Honorary Consultant Physician
University College London Medical School
London, UK

**WILEY-BLACKWELL**

A John Wiley & Sons, Ltd., Publication

BMJ|Books

This edition first published 2012 © 2012 by Blackwell Publishing Ltd.

BMJ Books is an imprint of BMJ Publishing Group Limited, used under licence by Blackwell Publishing which was acquired by John Wiley & Sons in February 2007. Blackwell's publishing programme has been merged with Wiley's global Scientific, Technical and Medical business to form Wiley-Blackwell.

*Registered office:* John Wiley & Sons, Ltd, The Atrium, Southern Gate, Chichester, West Sussex, PO19 8SQ, UK

*Editorial offices:* 9600 Garsington Road, Oxford, OX4 2DQ, UK

The Atrium, Southern Gate, Chichester, West Sussex, PO19 8SQ, UK

111 River Street, Hoboken, NJ 07030-5774, USA

For details of our global editorial offices, for customer services and for information about how to apply for permission to reuse the copyright material in this book please see our website at www.wiley.com/wiley-blackwell

The right of the author to be identified as the author of this work has been asserted in accordance with the UK Copyright, Designs and Patents Act 1988.

First published 1987
Second edition 1991
Third edition 1993
Fourth edition 1997
Fifth edition 2001

*Library of Congress Cataloging-in-Publication Data*
ABC of HIV and AIDS / edited by Michael W. Adler . . . [et al.]. – 6th ed.
    p. ; cm. – (ABC series)
  Rev. ed. of: ABC of AIDS / edited by Michael W. Adler. 5th ed. 2001.
  Includes bibliographical references and index.
  ISBN 978-1-4051-5700-1 (pbk. : alk. paper)
  I. Adler, Michael W. II. ABC of AIDS. III. Series: ABC series (Malden, Mass.)
  [DNLM: 1. Acquired Immunodeficiency Syndrome. 2. AIDS-Related Opportunistic Infections. 3. HIV Infections. WC 503]
  616.97′92–dc23

                                                                    2011049093

A catalogue record for this book is available from the British Library.

Wiley also publishes its books in a variety of electronic formats. Some content that appears in print may not be available in electronic books.

Set in 9.25/12 Minion by Laserwords Private Limited, Chennai, India
Printed and bound in Malaysia by Vivar Printing Sdn Bhd

1   2012

# Contents

# Contributors

**Michael W. Adler**

Emeritus Professor of Genitourinary Medicine/Sexually Transmitted Diseases, University College London Medical School, London, UK

**David Asboe**

Consultant Physician, Chelsea and Westminster Hospital, London, UK

**Paul Benn**

Consultant Physician, Mortimer Market Centre, London, UK

**John Booth**

Specialty Registrar in Nephrology, University College London Centre for Nephrology, Royal Free Hospital, London, UK

**Mark Bower**

Professor, Department of Oncology, Chelsea and Westminster Hospital, London, UK

**Ronan Breen**

Consultant Physician, Guy's and St Thomas' Hospital, London, UK

**Garry Brough**

Bloomsbury Clinic, Mortimer Market Centre, London, UK

**John Connolly**

Consultant Nephrologist and Honorary Senior Lecturer, Royal Free Hospital, London, UK

**Sarah Doffman**

Consultant Respiratory Physician, Brighton and Sussex University Hospitals NHS Trust, Royal Sussex County Hospital, Brighton, UK

**Simon G. Edwards**

Consultant GU/HIV Physician, Camden Provider Services, Mortimer Market Centre, London, UK

**Emma Fox**

Consultant Physician in Genitourinary Medicine, Kent Community Health Trust, Gate Clinic, Kent and Canterbury Hospital, Canterbury, UK

**Patrick French**

Consultant Physician in Genitourinary Medicine, Mortimer Market Centre, London, UK

**Brian Gazzard**

Professor, Imperial College London, London, UK

**Anna Maria Geretti**

Professor of Virology, Institute of Infection & Global Health, University of Liverpool, London, UK

**Richard Gilson**

Senior Clinical Lecturer, Centre for Sexual Health and HIV Research, University College London, London, UK

**Graham J. Hart**

Professor, Director of the Division of Population Health, Faculty of Biomedical Sciences, Centre for Sexual Health and HIV Research, University College London, London, UK

**Barbara Hedge**

Head of Psychology, St Helens and Knowsley Teaching Hospitals NHS Trust, Merseyside, UK

**Elisabeth Higgins**

Consultant, Department of Dermatology, Kings College Hospital, London, UK

**John Imrie**

Assistant Director, Africa Centre for Health and Population Studies, University of KwaZulu-Natal, Somkhele, South Africa; Principal Research Associate, Centre for Sexual Health and HIV Research, University College London, London, UK

**Sue Lightman**

Professor of Clinical Ophthalmology, Moorfields Eye Hospital, London, UK

**Marc Lipman**

Senior Lecturer, Royal Free Hospital, University College London, London, UK

**Namatovu Lubega**

Patient Representative, London, UK

**William Lynn**

Consultant Physician in Infectious Diseases, Ealing Hospital, London, UK

**Hadi Manji**
Consultant Physician, National Hospital for Neurology, Queen Square, London, UK

**Paddy McMaster**
Consultant in Paediatric Infectious Diseases, North Manchester General Hospital, Manchester, UK

**Danielle Mercey**
Consultant Physician in Genitourinary Medicine, Central and North West London NHS Foundation Trust, London, UK

**Robert F. Miller**
Professor, Reader in Clinical Infection and Honorary Consultant Physician, University College London Medical School, London, UK

**Adrian Mindel**
Professor and Head of STI Research Centre, Westmead Hospital, Westmead, Sydney, NSW, Australia

**June Minton**
Lead Pharmacist HIV/GUM and Infectious Diseases, University College London Hospitals NHS Foundation Trust, Mortimer Market Centre, London, UK

**Rachael Morris-Jones**
Consultant Dermatologist, Department of Dermatology, Kings College Hospital, London, UK

**Mark Nelson**
Consultant Physician, Chelsea and Westminster Hospital, London; Senior Lecturer, Imperial College London, London, UK

**Mahdad Noursadeghi**
Senior Lecturer, University College London, Honorary Consultant University College Hospital, London, UK

**Adrian Palfreeman**
Consultant, University Hospitals of Leicester, Leicester, UK

**Felicity Perrin**
Consultant Physician, King's College Hospital, London, UK

**Deenan Pillay**
Professor of Virology, University College London; Honorary Consultant Virologist at University College London Hospital, University College London, London, UK

**Huw Price**
Clinical Research Fellow, University College London, London, UK

**Chris Sandford**
Patient Representative, Mortimer Market Centre, London, UK

**Gulshan Sethi**
Consultant Physician in Sexual Health and HIV, Department of Sexual Health, Guy's and St Thomas' NHS Foundation Trust, London, UK

**Suzy Stokes**
Emergency Medicine Trainee, Oxfordshire Deanery, UK

**Binta Sultan**
Academic Clinical Fellow in HIV and GU Medicine, University College London, Mortimer Market Centre, London, UK

**Melinda Tenant-Flowers**
Consultant in GU and HIV Medicine at King's College Hospital, Honorary Senior Lecturer at King's College London Medical School, London, UK

**Paola Vitiello**
Research Assistant, Department of Virology, University College London Royal Free Hospital, London, UK

**Laura Waters**
Consultant Physician, Mortimer Market Centre, London, UK

**Chris Wilkinson**
Lead Consultant in Sexual and Reproductive Healthcare, Central and North West London NHS Foundation Trust, Margaret Pyke Centre, London, UK

**Ian G. Williams**
Senior Lecturer and Honorary Consultant Physician, University College London Medical School, London, UK

**Christine Younan**
Clinical Fellow, Moorfields Eye Hospital, London UK and Consultant Ophthalmologist, Westmead and Sydney Eye Hospitals, Sydney, Australia

# Preface

It is now over 30 years since the first recognized cases of AIDS were reported in the USA. There are estimated to be over 30 million persons living with HIV worldwide. Closer to home, the Health Protection Agency estimated that the number of individuals living with HIV in the UK will exceed 100 000 for the first time in 2012. There have been major advances in HIV therapy and where access to appropriate treatment and care is available, the clinical picture has evolved from a terminal illness to a manageable life-long chronic condition. In resource rich settings the major cause of death is due to the sequelae of late diagnosis. In the UK, it is estimated that a quarter of individuals with HIV are unaware of their infection. In addition, approximately half continue to be diagnosed with HIV at a late stage of infection. Early diagnosis of HIV is paramount, delivering both individual health gains, i.e. prevention of opportunistic infections with associated morbidity and mortality, and public health benefits in the prevention of HIV transmission through behaviour modification.

Following HIV diagnosis in the UK, we can be reassured that the quality of HIV care received is high. Based on London data, 80% of newly diagnosed patients were seen in an HIV clinic within 1 month of diagnosis; 90% had an undetectable viral load (less than 50 copies/mL) 1 year after starting therapy; and 93% of those in care for more than a year had a CD4 count above 200 cells per $mm^3$. Antiretroviral regimens have become more convenient to take with the advent of coformulated medications and greater tolerability. HIV-infected patients spend most of their time out of hospital and in the community. It is likely that primary care will play a greater role in the testing and subsequent management of HIV-infected individuals.

The aim of the sixth edition of the *ABC of HIV/AIDS* is to provide those healthcare professionals not routinely dealing with HIV-infected patients to develop an up-to-date knowledge base and feel more skilled and comfortable about caring for these patients.

This revised edition not only contains updated chapters but has new sections which reflect the latest recommendations on HIV testing, routine monitoring, antiretroviral treatment and the patient's perspective.

# CHAPTER 1

# Development of the Epidemic

*B. Sultan[1] and M. W. Adler[2]*

[1]University College London, Mortimer Market Centre, London, UK
[2]University College London Medical School, London, UK

---

**OVERVIEW**

- The commonest mode of transmission of the virus is through sexual intercourse
- The growth of the epidemic has appeared to stabilize
- HIV continues to exhort a huge public health and economic burden
- In 2009, there were 33.3 million people living with HIV worldwide
- Sub-Saharan Africa has experienced a disproportionate burden of the global HIV epidemic
- 10 million people who are eligible for treatment under World Health Organization guidelines are still in need of treatment

---

## Development of the epidemic (Boxes 1.1 and 1.2)

The first recognized cases of the acquired immune deficiency syndrome (AIDS) occurred in the summer of 1981 in the USA. Reports began to appear of *Pneumocystis carinii* (now known as *jirovecii*) pneumonia and Kaposi sarcoma in young men, who it was subsequently realized were both homosexual and immunocompromised. Even though the condition became known early on as AIDS, its cause and modes of transmission were not immediately obvious. The virus, human immunodeficiency virus (HIV), now known to cause AIDS in a proportion of those infected, was discovered in 1983. Subsequently a new variant has been isolated in patients with West African connections, HIV-2.

Thirty years on and with the introduction of combination antiretroviral therapy (cART), where it is widely available, the clinical picture of HIV has changed from a fatal illness to that of a chronic condition. There has been an increase in the number of people living with diagnosed HIV as a result of fewer deaths from AIDS and ongoing high rates of HIV diagnosis. In developed countries, where cART has been available from its inception, an ageing cohort is now seen, and people with HIV are living near-normal life expectancies. Consequent to this has arisen the challenges of managing the co-morbidities associated with age and the long-term consequences of cART. Despite this, more than 10 million people worldwide who require cART are not able to access it, and HIV continues to exhort a huge public health and economic burden. The last decade has seen consistent global efforts to address health, development and the HIV epidemic, starting with the United Nations (UN) Millennium Development Goals (MDGs). Despite extensive progress, many countries have failed to achieve MDG Six, which is in part to halt and reverse the spread of HIV (Box 1.2)

---

Box 1.1 **Early history of the HIV epidemic**

- 1981 Cases of *Pneumocystis carinii* pneumonia and Kaposi sarcoma in the USA
- 1983 Virus discovered
- 1984 Development of the antibody test
- 1987 Introduction of zidovudine therapy
- 1995 Formation of United Nations Programme on AIDS (UNAIDS)
- 1996 Introduction of highly active antiretroviral therapy (HAART)
- 2003 The '3 by 5' campaign is launched to widen access to treatment

---

Box 1.2 **HIV epidemic – the bottom line**

UN Millennium Development Goal Six

- Target **6A**. Have halted by 2015 and begun to reverse the spread of HIV/AIDS
- Target **6B**. Achieve, by 2010, universal access to treatment for HIV/AIDS for all those who need it.

'Growth in investment for the AIDS response has flattened for the first time in 2009. Stigma, discrimination, and bad laws continue to place roadblocks for people living with HIV and people on the margins . . . . This new fourth decade of the epidemic should be one of moving towards efficient, focused and scaled-up programmes to accelerate progress for Results. Results. Results'

Michel Sidibé, Executive Director UNAIDS, UNAIDS Report on the Global AIDS Epidemic 2010

---

*ABC of HIV and AIDS*, Sixth Edition. Edited by Michael W. Adler,
Simon G. Edwards, Robert F. Miller, Gulshan Sethi and Ian G. Williams.
© 2012 Blackwell Publishing Ltd. Published 2012 by Blackwell Publishing Ltd.

## Transmission of the virus (Box 1.3)

HIV has been isolated from semen, cervical secretions, lymphocytes, cell-free plasma, cerebrospinal fluid, tears, saliva, urine and breast milk. This does not mean, however, that these fluids all transmit infection, as the concentration of virus in them varies considerably.

---

Box 1.3 **Transmission of the virus**

Sexual intercourse
- anal
- vaginal
- oral

Contaminated needles
- intravenous drug users
- needlestick injuries

Mother to child
- *in utero*
- at birth
- breastfeeding

Tissue donation
- blood transfusion
- organ transplantation

---

Particularly infectious are semen, blood and possibly cervical secretions. Infection can occur after mucosal exposure to infected blood or body fluids.

The commonest mode of transmission of the virus throughout the world is through sexual intercourse. Unprotected anal and vaginal intercourse carry the highest risk of transmission, and the promotion of condom use has been the focus of prevention efforts.

Transmission also occurs through the sharing or reuse of contaminated needles by injecting drug users, which continues to drive the epidemic in Eastern Europe.

Transmission from mother to child occurs *in utero*, during labour and through breastfeeding. Transmission rates can be between 15%

and 45% without intervention, and less than 5% with effective interventions. Mother-to-child transmission (MTCT) of HIV still significantly contributes to child mortality worldwide. However, the increase in access to services for preventing MTCT has led to fewer children being born with HIV. Use of cART during pregnancy, and at the time of birth, has been the mainstay of intervention strategies (see Chapters 17 and 18). In the UK, universal antenatal screening and access to cART have virtually eliminated MTCT. Globally, an estimated 370 000 children were newly infected with HIV in 2007, a fall of 24% from 5 years previously. UNAIDS called for the elimination of new paediatric HIV infections by 2015. It recommends that countries adopt a policy that HIV-positive mothers or their infants take ART while breastfeeding to prevent HIV transmission.

Contaminated blood products have previously contributed to the transmission of HIV, but universal screening has almost eliminated this mode of transmission in developed countries. Healthcare workers can rarely be infected through needlestick injuries and skin and mucosal exposure to infected blood or body fluids.

## Growth and size of the epidemic (Table 1.1, Figure 1.1)

The growth of the epidemic has appeared to stabilize. Globally, there are fewer AIDS-related deaths and a steady decline in the number of new HIV infections since the late 1990s. In 2009, there were 33.3 million people living with HIV. There were 2.6 million new infections, which is 21% fewer than in 1997 (3.2 million) when the number of new infections reached its peak. HIV remains undiagnosed in 40% of people. The HIV incidence in 33 countries has fallen by 25% between 2001 and 2009, with 22 of these countries being in sub-Saharan Africa. However, in seven countries there has been an increase of more than 25% in the same time period. These include five countries in Eastern Europe and Central Asia.

Even though North America and Europe experienced the first impact of the epidemic, infections with HIV are now seen throughout the world, and the major focus of the epidemic is in resource-poor countries.

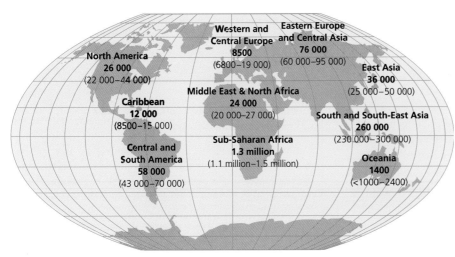

**Total: 1.8 million** (1.6 million–2.1 million)

**Figure 1.1** Estimated adult and child deaths from AIDS, 2009. *Source:* UNAIDS, UNAIDS Report on the Global AIDS Epidemic 2010.

**Table 1.1**  Regional HIV and AIDS statistics 2009.

|  | Adults and children living with HIV | Adults and children newly infected with HIV | Adult prevalence (15–49 years) (%) | Adult & child deaths due to AIDS |
|---|---|---|---|---|
| Sub-Saharan Africa | 22.5 million (20.9 million–24.2 million) | 1.8 million (1.6 million–2.0 million) | 5.0 (4.7–5.2) | 1.3 million (1.1 million–1.5 million) |
| Middle East and North Africa | 460 000 (400 000–530 000) | 75 000 (61 000–92 000) | 0.2 (0.2–0.3) | 24 000 (20 000–27 000) |
| South and South-East Asia | 4.1 million (3.7 million–4.6 million) | 270 000 (240 000–320 000) | 0.3 (0.3–0.3) | 260 000 (230 000–300 000) |
| East Asia | 770 000 (560 000–1.0 million) | 82 000 (48 000–140 000) | 0.1 (0.1–0.1) | 36 000 (25 000–50 000) |
| Central and South America | 1.4 million (1.2 million–1.6 million) | 92 000 (70 000–120 000) | 0.5 (0.4–0.6) | 58 000 (43 000–70 000) |
| Caribbean | 240 000 (220 000–270 000) | 17 000 (13 000–21 000) | 1.0 (0.9–1.1) | 12 000 (8500–15 000) |
| Eastern Europe and Central Asia | 1.4 million (1.3 million–1.6 million) | 130 000 (110 000–160 000) | 0.8 (0.7–0.9) | 76 000 (60 000–95 000) |
| Western and Central Europe | 820 000 (720 000–910 000) | 31 000 (23 000–40 000) | 0.2 (0.2–0.2) | 8500 (6800–19 000) |
| North America | 1.5 million (1.2 million–2.0 million) | 70 000 (44 000–130 000) | 0.5 (0.4–0.7) | 26 000 (22 000–44 000) |
| Oceania | 57 000 (50 000–64 000) | 4500 (3400–6000) | 0.3 (0.2–0.3) | 1400 (<1000–2400) |
| Total | 33.3 million (31.4 million–35.3 million) | 2.6 million (2.3 million–2.8 million) | 0.8 (0.7–0.8) | 1.8 million (1.6 million–2.1 million) |

The ranges around the estimates in this table define the boundaries within which the actual numbers lie, based on the best available information.
*Source:* UNAIDS Report on the Global AIDS Epidemic 2010.

## UK, Western Europe and USA

The number of people living with HIV in North America and Western and Central Europe has increased, with a 30% rise since 2001, and reached an estimated 2.3 million people in 2009. Heterosexual transmission represents about 50% of new HIV infections. In 2007, almost 17% of these new infections were among people from countries with generalized epidemics. The data are indicative of a resurgence of the HIV epidemic among men who have sex with men (MSM) in North America and Western Europe. Between 2000 and 2006 there was an 86% rise in the annual number of new HIV diagnoses in this risk group.

In the UK, the Health protection Agency (HPA) predicts that by 2012 the number of people living with HIV will continue to rise and reach 100 000. In 2009 there was an estimated 86 500 people thought to be living with HIV, 26% of these with undiagnosed infections. Among those with diagnosed HIV, 43% are MSM, 51% are heterosexuals and 2% are injecting drug users (Table 1.2).

In 2010, the largest number of new diagnoses of HIV in the UK was recorded among MSM (Figure 1.2). Most infections among heterosexuals were acquired abroad, the majority from sub-Saharan Africa. There is a downward trend in the numbers of infections acquired abroad, thought to be due in part to changes in immigration policies (Figure 1.3).

In the USA there were an estimated 1,099,161 people living with HIV by the end of 2009 (Table 1.2), 48% among MSM, 25% in injecting drug users and 18% in heterosexuals. HIV disproportionately affects racial and ethnic minorities, with 45% of newly infected people in 2006 arising from the African-American population.

**Table 1.2**  Cumulative reported cases of diagnosed HIV by exposure category in the USA and UK, 2009.

| Exposure category | USA* | Proportion (%) | UK† | Proportion |
|---|---|---|---|---|
| Men who have sex with men (MSM) | 529 908 | 48 | 28 090 | 43 |
| Injecting drug use (IDU) | 273 444 | 25 | 1550 | 2 |
| MSM/DU | 77 213 | 7 |  |  |
| Heterosexual | 198 820 | 18 | 33 310 | 51 |
| Other | 19 776 | 2 | 2369 | 4 |
| **Total** | **1 099 161** | **100** | **65 319** | **100** |

*Centre for Disease Control (CDC), USA.
†Health Protection Agency (HPA), UK.

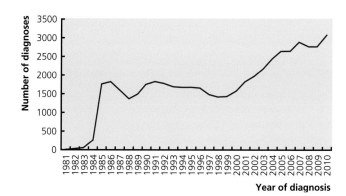

**Figure 1.2**  Annual New HIV diagnoses among men who have sex with men, UK, 1981–2010. *Source:* Health Protection Agency.

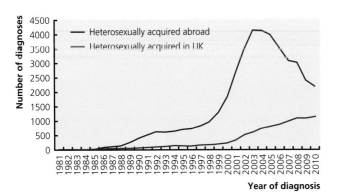

**Figure 1.3** Annual New HIV diagnoses acquired heterosexually, UK, 1981–2010. *Source:* Health Protection Agency.

## Worldwide

In the developing world, HIV is spread mainly through heterosexual intercourse. The epidemic in this region has been driven by a combination of poor economies and an absence of functioning health systems leading to lack of access to early diagnosis and cART.

## Africa

Sub-Saharan Africa has experienced a disproportionate burden of the global HIV epidemic (Box 1.4). In 2009, 22.5 million people were living with HIV in this region, accounting for 68% of the global total. Swaziland has the highest adult prevalence of HIV in the world, with an estimate of 25.9%. Southern Africa is still the most affected by the HIV epidemic, with an estimated 11.3 million people living with HIV in 2009, an increase of more than 30% in 10 years. South Africa's epidemic remains the largest in the world (Box 1.5). However, there is an indication of slowing of HIV incidence in Southern Africa as well as in East Africa. The HIV prevalence in Kenya fell from 14% in the mid-1990s to 5% in 2006.

---

**Box 1.4 HIV/AIDS epidemic disproportionality**

- >**50%** of people with HIV are **women or girls**
- **68%** of people with HIV live in **sub-Saharan Africa**
- **Young women** aged 15–24 years are **eight times** more likely than men to have HIV in sub-Saharan Africa
- **34 million** children have been orphaned overall
- **80%** of all the world's children orphaned by HIV/AIDS reside in **sub-Saharan Africa**

---

**Box 1.5 South Africa's epidemic**

- 5.6 million people living with HIV
- 1 in 3 women aged 30–34 living with HIV
- 1 in 4 men aged 30–39 living with HIV
- Life expectancy now less than 50 years in three provinces

---

## Central and South America

There has been little change in the HIV epidemic in Central and South America, with an estimated 1.4 million people living with HIV. One third of those affected live in Brazil. The HIV rates in this region have been contained largely by the availability of cART and early HIV prevention and treatment strategies.

## Asia

The epidemic in Asia is stable, with an estimated 4.9 million persons living with HIV in 2009. Thailand has the highest prevalence in the region, with a prevalence of 1%. The HIV prevalence is increasing in Pakistan, Bangladesh and the Philippines, but still remains low in these countries. There was a 25% decrease in HIV incidence in India and Nepal between 2001 and 2009. There are wide variations in the epidemic in Asia, both within and between countries and risk groups. For example, in China, five out of 22 provinces account for more than 50% of people living with HIV.

## Eastern Europe and Central Asia

There has been an almost threefold increase between 2001 and 2009 in the number of people living with HIV in Eastern Europe and Central Asia, with an estimate of 1.4 million in 2009. The Russian Federation and the Ukraine account for 90% of these people with new HIV diagnoses. The epidemic in this region has been driven mostly by infections among injecting drug users, sex workers and their partners. An estimated 37% of people who inject drugs in the Russian Federation are thought to have HIV, with estimates in the Ukraine ranging from 39% to 50%. The upward trend continues, and the interaction between injecting drug use and sex work is fuelling the epidemic in this region.

## Public health and policy

National policies have influenced the HIV epidemic in certain regions. Needle exchange programmes are an effective strategy to prevent onward transmission of HIV among injecting drug users and have been adopted in many countries. However, in others, such as the Russian Federation, there is a lack of political will to implement these programmes, with only an estimated 7% of injecting drug users able to access needle exchange programmes, which are mostly run by non-governmental organizations. This situation is reflected across most of Eastern Europe and Central Asia, and has contributed to the rise in the number of HIV infections in this region.

Immigration policy can also influence the nature of regional epidemics. In the UK, for example, the fall in the number of new HIV infections acquired abroad amongst heterosexuals since 2002 has been in part due to the change in UK immigration policy to immigrants from sub-Saharan Africa.

## Future

The HIV epidemic has had a profound influence on the economic and political structures of many developing countries, particularly in sub-Saharan Africa (Box 1.6). The UNAIDS estimates that in 2010 there were approximately 20 million children in sub-Saharan Africa who had lost at least one parent to AIDS. This not only represents a breakdown in family structure but also the loss of a whole generation of young working adults, resulting in devastating consequences for already struggling economies. Population growth and death rates are increasingly affected. Countries with an adult prevalence of over 10% are expected to see an average reduction in life expectancy of 17 years by 2015.

---

Box 1.6 **Economic Consequences of HIV/AIDS**

- ↓Economic growth 2–4% across sub-Saharan Africa
- ↓GDP 1% per year in countries with 15–20% prevalence rates
- ↓GDP 17% South Africa by 2010
- ↓Indian economic growth by 0.86% per year

*Source:* World Health Organization (WHO) Trade, foreign policy, diplomacy and health: HIV and AIDS. http://www.who.int/trade/glossary/story051/en/index.htm.

---

Despite these large numbers there has been a decline in people with new HIV infections, in large part due to public health efforts of health promotion and education strategies, such as condom use and addressing the issue of concurrent partners, as well as the availability

---

Box 1.7 **Treatment 2.0, UNAIDS, 2011**

To achieve the full benefits of Treatment 2.0 progress has to be made across five areas:

1 **Create a better pill and diagnostics:** UNAIDS calls for the innovation of a smarter, better pill that is less toxic and for diagnostics that are easier to use. A simple diagnostic tool could help to reduce the burden on health systems.
2 **Treatment as prevention:** antiretroviral therapy reduces the level of the virus in the body. Evidence shows that when people living with HIV have lowered their viral load they are less likely to transmit HIV.
3 **Stop cost being an obstacle:** despite drastic reductions in drug pricing over the past ten years, the costs of antiretroviral therapy programmes continue to rise. Drugs can be even more affordable – however, potential gains are highest in the area of reducing the non-drug-related costs of providing treatment. Treatment 2.0 is expected to reduce the cost per AIDS-related death averted by half.
4 **Improve uptake of voluntary HIV testing and counselling and linkages to care**: when people know their HIV status they can start treatment when their CD4 count is around 350 cells/μL. Starting treatment at the right time increases the efficacy of current treatment regimens and increases life expectancy.
5 **Strengthen community mobilization**: by involving the community in managing treatment programmes, treatment access and adherence can be improved. Demand creation will also help bring down costs for extensive outreach and help reduce the burden on health care system.

---

of cART. In South Africa there are indications of a paradigm shift towards safer sex among young people. In Zimbabwe there are proportionally fewer men with casual partners and there is higher condom use between regular partners.

Treatment 2.0 (Box 1.7) is a new approach from UNAIDS and its partners to simplify the way HIV treatment is provided and to scale-up access to medicines. Mathematical modelling suggests that Treatment 2.0 could avert an additional 10 million deaths by 2025, compared to current strategies.

Globally, more than 5 million people are receiving HIV treatment. Since 2004 there has been a 13-fold increase in the number of people receiving cART, representing more than 5 million people. Access to cART is thought to have contributed to a 19% decrease in deaths among those with HIV. However, 10 million people who are eligible for treatment under WHO guidelines are still in need of treatment, the majority of whom are in developing countries. Forty per cent of people with HIV are undiagnosed, resulting in presentation at a late stage in the disease course and poorer outcomes. This is in part due to inadequate healthcare systems and persistent stigma in many countries, particularly those in Africa.

National and international policy efforts need to be redoubled to ensure there is access to early diagnosis and treatment. Political and health infrastructures need to be strengthened to deliver public health messages and much needed healthcare. These are essential to controlling and reversing the trend of the current HIV epidemic.

## Acknowledgement

The data on AIDS/HIV is reproduced with permission from the Health Protection Agency and the United Nations AIDS Programme.

## Further reading

UNAIDS. UNAIDS Report on the Global AIDS Epidemic 2010. (www.unaids.org/globalreport/Global_report.htm).

UNAIDS. UNAIDS in 2011. (www.unaids.org/en/resources/presscentre/featurestories/2010/december/20101230unaidsin2011).

WHO. HIV/AIDS. (www.who.int/topics/hiv_aids/en).

Centre for Disease Control and Prevention (CDC). HIV/AIDS Statistics and Surveillance. (www.cdc.gov/hiv/topics/surveillance/index.htm).

Health Protection Agency (HPA). HIV in the United Kingdom, Report 2010. (www.hpa.org.uk/web/HPAweb&HPAwebStandard/HPAweb_C/1287145264558).

Mathers BM, Degenhardt L, Ali H, *et al.* for the 2009 Reference Group to the UN on HIV and Injecting Drug Use. HIV prevention, treatment and care services for people who inject drugs: a systematic review of global, regional, and national coverage. *Lancet* 2010;375:1014–1028.

# CHAPTER 2

# Immunology of HIV-1 Infection

*M. Noursadeghi and D. Pillay*

University College London, London, UK

## OVERVIEW

- During transmission of infection, HIV-1 interacts with macrophages and dendritic cells at the site of inoculation, leading to transfer of virus to CD4 T cells within lymph nodes, where the majority of viral replication occurs
- HIV-1 replication induces antiviral antibody and cytotoxic T-cell responses that help to control HIV replication during primary infection
- HIV-1 displays various mechanisms of immune evasion that help to prevent its eradication despite antiviral immune responses
- HIV-1 induces widespread dysregulated immune activation that causes depletion of circulating CD4 T cells by sequestration of memory T cells within lymph nodes and exhaustion of the naïve T-cell pool
- Immunodeficiency in AIDS is due to multiple mechanisms, including abnormalities of macrophage, dendritic cell, B cell and CD8 T-cell function as well the effects on CD4 T cells

## Introduction

The interactions of HIV-1 with the immune system contribute extensively to the pathogenesis of AIDS. These interactions are critical during HIV-1 transmission. They also largely determine the rate of progression from primary HIV infection to AIDS, and underlie multiple mechanisms for the immunodeficiency that ensues. An understanding of the immunology of HIV-1 informs our current clinical management of patients with AIDS and fuels the development of novel strategies for prevention and treatment of HIV-1 infection or AIDS-related disease.

## Primary infection

HIV-1 targets several different cells of the human immune system, principally through interaction of the HIV-1 envelope glycoprotein, gp120, with two host cell surface receptors, CD4 and a chemokine receptor. CD4 is an important co-receptor for T cells involved

in T-cell receptor recognition of exogenous antigens presented by major histocompatibility complex (MHC) class II molecules. Chemokines comprise a large family of soluble mediators that regulate movement of cells within the immune system. HIV-1 interacts variably with one of two chemokine receptors, called CXCR4 and CCR5. Chemokine receptor selectivity is determined by variable regions in gp120 that render HIV-1 strains tropic for either CXCR4, CCR5 or dual tropic. Both CXCR4 and CCR5 are expressed by CD4 T cells. CCR5 is also expressed by tissue macrophages and dendritic cells.

The majority of HIV-1 infection *in vivo* exists within CD4 T cells. There is also evidence for HIV-1 infection within tissue macrophages. There is less evidence for active HIV-1 replication within dendritic cells. Importantly, however, dendritic cells can also capture HIV-1 via a $Ca^{2+}$-dependent lectin receptor called DC-SIGN. This does not trigger HIV-1 fusion and integration, but rather endocytosis of virus that is subsequently displayed at the cell surface (see Figure 2.3b). Importantly the interaction of DC-SIGN with HIV-1 stimulates so-called maturation and migration of dendritic cells to regional lymph nodes where HIV-1 on the surface of dendritic cells will encounter permissive CD4 T cells.

The current paradigm for the natural route of primary HIV-1 infection via mucosal surfaces therefore proposes that resident macrophages and dendritic cells may be the primary host cells targeted by HIV-1. They then propagate transmission of HIV-1 to T cells that are recruited locally or within regional lymph nodes (Figure 2.1). This model is supported by a variety of observations. Sexual HIV-1 transmission is significantly associated with concurrent inflammatory conditions of the recipient mucosa in which HIV-permissive macrophages and dendritic cells may be more abundant. In addition, HIV-1 strains isolated during primary infection are predominantly CCR5 or macrophage tropic, and CCR5-deficient individuals are relatively resistant to HIV-1 infection. Recent studies on HIV-1 founder viruses that establish successful infection confirm that these viruses are CCR5 tropic, but surprisingly unable to infect macrophages, suggesting that local T cells may in fact form the first founder population of infected cells.

## Antiviral host immune responses

The seroconversion illness that follows primary infection with HIV-1 coincides with a transient peak of viral replication. Patients'

*ABC of HIV and AIDS*, Sixth Edition. Edited by Michael W. Adler,
Simon G. Edwards, Robert F. Miller, Gulshan Sethi and Ian G. Williams.
© 2012 Blackwell Publishing Ltd. Published 2012 by Blackwell Publishing Ltd.

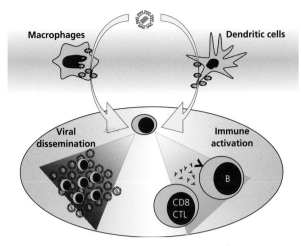

**Figure 2.1** Primary HIV-1 infection. HIV-1 initially infects macrophages or is captured by DC-SIGN on dendritic cells at the site of mucosal inoculation. The virus is then passaged through these cells and transferred to CD4 T cells in regional (draining) lymph nodes, where it rapidly replicates. Viral replication concurrently stimulates antiviral antibody and cytotoxic T-cell immune responses that help to control the initial viraemia associated with primary infection.

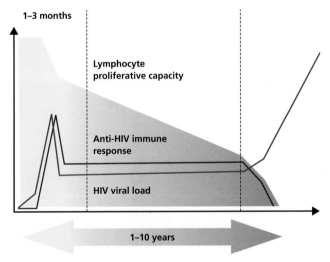

**Figure 2.2** The relationship between HIV-1 replication and anti-HIV responses during progressive HIV-1 infection. Anti-HIV immune responses control the initial burst of viral replication after primary infection but do not eradicate the virus. Instead active viral replication and the consequent antiviral response establish a homeostatic set point that may persist for many years. During this time, ongoing viral replication and dysregulated immune stimulation deplete the host's lymphocyte proliferative capacity, until eventually the antiviral response cannot be maintained and viral replication increases.

symptoms and the fall in HIV-1 viral load is ascribed to the antiviral host immune response (Figure 2.2). Non-specific (innate) interferon and specific (adaptive) humoral (antibody) and cellular immune responses to HIV-1 can be readily demonstrated at this time.

The cellular adaptive immune response to viral pathogens is principally mediated by CD8 cytotoxic T lymphocytes (CTLs) that recognize antigens presented by MHC class I at the surface of infected host cells. CTLs kill virus-infected cells by causing cell lysis.

In most cases three or four separate CTL clones can be demonstrated that recognize different HIV-1 epitopes. During primary infection. the appearance of CTLs correlate temporally and quantitatively with the fall in HIV-1 viral load. Furthermore, greater numbers of CTLs and a broader repertoire of CTL clones both correlate with delay in disease progression and the onset of AIDS. The role of interferon (IFN) and antibody responses in the control of viraemia during primary HIV infection is less clear.

## HIV-1 evasion of host immunity

Although IFN, antibody and CTL responses to HIV-1 may contribute to the initial control of HIV-1 viral load after primary infection, they do not establish sterilizing immunity. Viral replication continues and eventually overwhelms the immune response as patients develop AIDS. Immunological evasion underlies the ability of HIV-1 to cause persistent infection, avoid the development of natural protective immunity and resist extensive efforts to produce a protective vaccination strategy. Numerous mechanisms have been identified by which HIV-1 can evade the host immune system.

Protective antibodies are required to recognize the HIV-1 envelope. Anti-gp120 antibodies are produced by all patients, but *in vivo*, these antibodies are non-neutralizing, meaning that they are unable to clear the virus or prevent infection after vaccination. This is partly because gp120 associates with another glycoprotein, called gp41, in trimeric complexes that form spikes in the surface membrane of the virus (Figure 2.3a). The immunodominant epitopes are hidden within the core of these complexes and therefore inaccessible to antibodies. Heavy glycosylation of gp120 also has the effect of inhibiting antibody binding.

The error-prone nature of HIV-1 reverse transcriptase activity during viral replication is also a key factor in viral escape from host immune responses. New mutations appear in approximately one-third of the virus produced, such that every possible point mutation in the HIV-1 genome arises on a daily basis. This generates hypervariable regions in gp120 that are more abundant on the exposed surface of gp41–gp120 complexes and contribute to viral escape from antibodies.

The continuous generation of mutant virus also underpins HIV-1 escape from antiviral CTL responses. In order to elicit these responses, HIV-1 antigens must be presented by MHC class I molecules on the surface of infected cells. In population studies, HIV-1 virus sequences have been found to have changed such that they cannot be presented by the most effective MHC class I molecules. In addition, components of HIV-1, particularly the accessory protein nef, reduce MHC class I expression (Figure 2.3b), and the ability of HIV-1 to bind the receptor DC-SIGN on dendritic cells allows it to avoid the normal antigen processing pathway. All of these mechanisms serve to allow HIV-infected cells to go 'unnoticed'.

Innate immune defences are also undermined by HIV-1. IFN stimulates the expression of many genes that can 'restrict' the HIV-1 life cycle, but numerous mechanisms have been identified by which components of HIV-1 has evolved to avoid or degrade these defences. Finally, the ability for HIV-1 to establish latent infection, namely integrate into the host cell genome without replicating, is also an important immune evasion mechanism. During this

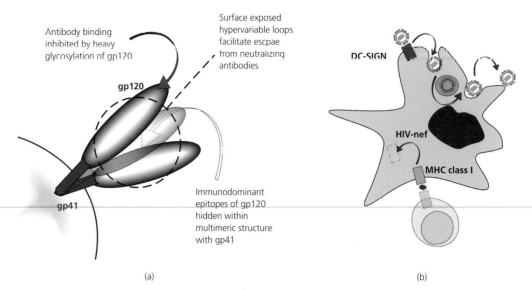

(a)

(b)

**Figure 2.3** Mechanisms of immune evasion by HIV-1. (a) Naturally occurring anti-gp120 antibodies are mostly non-neutralizing. Immunodominant epitopes for these antibodies are hidden in the core of the gp41–gp120 trimeric complex, and antibody binding is further inhibited by heavy glycosylation. In addition the exposed surface, gp120 has multiple hypervariable regions that facilitate viral escape from antibody-mediated immunity. (b) A number of mechanisms also reduce presentation of HIV-1 antigens by dendritic cells. Virus binding and internalization via DC-SIGN avoids the normal exogenous antigen processing pathway, and HIV accessory proteins such as nef reduce MHC class I surface expression and therefore presentation of the products of viral replication.

time viral genes are not expressed and therefore cannot induce an immune response. Latent infections typically occur in long-lived memory CD4 T cells and tissue macrophages which form persistent and long-lived virus reservoirs.

## Immunodeficiency

Progressive immunodeficiency and hence susceptibility to opportunistic infections or neoplasia is the hallmark of AIDS. The most widely used surrogate of immunodeficiency is destruction of naïve and memory CD4 T-cell populations.

Antigen naïve CD4 T cells recognize antigen presented with MHC class II by professional antigen-presenting cells. Clonal T-cell proliferation then follows, amplifying and regulating the wide spectrum of humoral and cellular immune responses. This process also leads to production of long-lived memory T cells with high affinity T-cell receptors for specific antigens that are primed to respond rapidly to subsequent antigenic challenge giving rise to the so-called recall antigen response.

During progressive HIV-1 infection and AIDS there is initially depletion of memory CD4 T cells followed by loss of naïve CD4 T cells. HIV-1 infection of CD4 T cells does cause cell lysis, but T-cell depletion seems to exceed the population apparently infected with virus. The mechanisms that contribute to T-cell loss are not yet fully understood, but the current paradigm suggests that HIV-1 replication occurs mainly within lymphoid tissues and causes immune activation (Figure 2.1). As discussed already, the consequent anti-viral immune responses partly control HIV-1 viral load, but since they do not eradicate the virus persistent viral replication and therefore persistent immune activation achieve a homeostatic set point (Figure 2.2). This corresponds to clinically asymptomatic state between primary HIV-1 infection and AIDS, which typically lasts 5–10 years, albeit with marked variability. This

phase may progress rapidly (less than 1 year) in some patients or last longer than 10 years in 'long-term non-progressor' patients.

Persistent immune activation by HIV-1 may contribute to T-cell loss by two principle mechanisms (Figure 2.4). The early reduction in memory CD4 T cells is thought to be due to sequestration within activated lymphoid tissue. The subsequent loss of naïve T cells is attributed to a finite capacity for cellular activation and proliferation. In this model, lymphopenia results from persistent HIV-1 replication that stimulates cellular activation, and consequently activation-induced cell death or apoptosis, until the available naïve

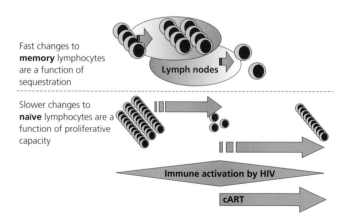

**Figure 2.4** Principle mechanisms for the changes to lymphocyte numbers during progressive HIV-1 infection and after cART. Dysregulated immune activation induced by HIV-1 depletes circulating lymphocyte by two main mechanisms. First by sequestration of memory cells within immunologically active lymphoid tissue and then by depletion of naïve cells by gradual exhaustion of the naïve cell pool. As immune activation is reduced by suppression of viral replication by cART recovery of memory cells is seen initially as they are released from sequestered sites, followed by much slower recovery of naïve cells as the lymphocyte proliferative capacity is gradually replenished.

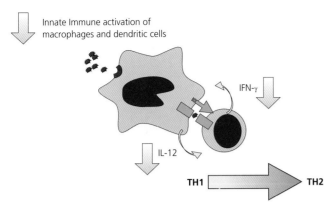

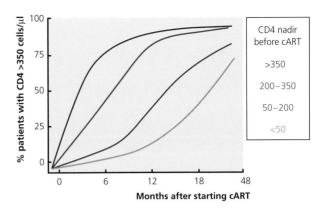

**Figure 2.5** Possible HIV-1 effects on macrophage and dendritic cell function. Innate immune activation of macrophages and dendritic cells promotes a so-called TH1 type adaptive immune response which supports the production of interferon (IFN)-γ and cell-mediated host defences that are critical for intracellular infection such as those caused by mycobacteria. HIV-1 infection is associated with reduced innate immune activation of macrophages and dendritic cells, and reduced interleukin (IL)-12 production by these cells. IL-12 being the main stimulus for TH1 responses, a bias towards TH2 type responses associated with diminished IFN-γ production in HIV-infected patients is reported and may contribute to immunodeficiency in AIDS.

**Figure 2.6** CD4 T-cell recovery after cART. The rate of recovery of circulating CD4 T-cell counts after cART is partly dependent on the CD4 nadir before starting cART. CD4 counts may continue to improve for several years in patients who had very low CD4 counts before starting treatment.

T cell pool is exhausted (Figure 2.2). This process is accelerated by a high rate of viral replication either as a result of poor anti-HIV immune responses, the generation of HIV-1 mutants that are able to evade host immunity and eventually by diminished ability of bone marrow progenitor cells to replenish the naïve T-cell pool. Another important mechanism for chronic immune activation and T-cell depletion focuses on HIV-1 replication in the gastrointestinal mucosa. This is thought to lead to early and substantial T-cell loss as a direct result of HIV-1 replication, and translocation of microbial products across the gut mucosal barrier that cause chronic immune activation and contribute further to systemic immune deficiency.

Importantly, HIV-1 does not simply induce anti-HIV responses but extensively dysregulated immune activation. This is illustrated by a variety of findings. T-cell proliferative responses to many stimuli become abnormal. Although quantitatively CD8 T-cell populations persist until very advanced HIV-1 disease, when all lymphocyte numbers fall, CD8 CTL function is impaired much earlier. B-cell hyperreactivity is also reflected in hypergammaglobulinaemia and bone marrow plasmacytosis, but is paradoxically associated with attenuated B-cell (antibody) responses to vaccination, suggesting impairment of specific B-cell function that mirrors the effects of HIV-1 on T cells.

Macrophage and dendritic cell dysfunction during HIV-1 infection are also recognized. These cells are involved in innate immune recognition of pathogens, early recruitment of host defences to the site of an infection and augmentation of adaptive immune responses. The effects of HIV-1 on these cells may therefore concurrently contribute to dysfunction of innate and adaptive immunity (Figure 2.5).

## The response to cART

Circulating CD4 T-cell counts rise following cART in most patients. This correlates strongly with the reduction in opportunistic infections in AIDS. The recovery of CD4 T cells is thought to result from reduction in HIV-driven dysregulated immune activation as viral replication is suppressed by cART (Figure 2.4). There is initially redistribution of lymph node-sequestered memory T cells, typically within 2 months. This is temporally associated with the development of immune reconstitution diseases in some patients with concurrent opportunistic infections. There is then gradual recovery of naïve T-cell populations that may continue over 2 years in patients who have had a very low CD4 T-cell nadir before starting cART (Figure 2.6). Recovery of CD4 T-cell activation markers, proliferation responses to recall antigens and T-cell receptor repertoires are also reported, but these seem to be incomplete. Limited studies also suggest only partial recovery of abnormal B-cell function after cART, and in some patients refractory reconstitution of the immune system has been associated with features that suggest persistent immune activation. A consensus view on the effect of cART on anti-HIV immune responses is not yet established, but most data suggest that HIV-specific responses decline as viral replication is suppressed. Rapid viral rebound during treatment interruptions confirm that the immune system is not able to control HIV replication after cART.

## Further reading

Battegay M, Nuesch R, Hirschel B, Kaufmann GR. Immunological recovery and antiretroviral therapy in HIV-1 infection. *Lancet Infect Dis* 2006;6: 280–287.

Brander C, Riviere Y. Early and late cytotoxic T lymphocyte responses in HIV infection. *AIDS* 2002;16(Suppl 4):S97–103.

Brenchley JM, Douek, DC. HIV infection and the gastrointestinal immune system. *Mucosal Immunol* 2008;1:23–30.

Haase AT. Early events in sexual transmission of HIV and SIV and opportunities for interventions. *Annu Rev Med* 2011;62:127–139.

Noursadeghi M, Katz DR, Miller RF. HIV-1 infection of mononuclear phagocytic cells: the case for bacterial innate immune deficiency in AIDS. *Lancet Infect Dis* 2006;6:794–804.

Pantophlet R, Burton DR. GP120: target for neutralizing HIV-1 Antibodies. *Annu Rev Immunol* 2006;24:739–769.

Peterlin BM, Trono D. Hide, shield and strike back: how HIV-infected cells avoid immune eradication. *Nat Rev Immunol* 2003;3:97–107.

# CHAPTER 3

# Viral Assays Used in the Diagnosis and Management of HIV Infection

*A. M. Geretti[1] and P. Vitiello[2]*

[1] Institute of Infection & Global Health, University of Liverpool, UK
[2] University College London, UK

## OVERVIEW

- The recommended first-line screening test for HIV infection is a laboratory assay that tests for HIV antibody and p24 antigen simultaneously. This is called a fourth-generation assay
- Rapid HIV diagnosis can be achieved within 30 minutes using a variety of point-of-care tests
- HIV RNA or proviral DNA testing is also used to diagnose vertical HIV transmission in newborns from HIV-positive mothers, as maternal HIV antibodies persist for up to 18 months, making serology results difficult to interpret
- The HIV-1 RNA load in plasma is a marker of infectiousness and a potent predictor of the rate of CD4 decline, disease progression and mortality. In patients on combination antiretroviral therapy (cART), the viral load provides the main surrogate marker for the clinical efficacy of cART
- Genotypic resistance testing identifies HIV strains resistant to antiretroviral drugs as the virus carries key mutations in the targets of cART. It should be performed prior to starting therapy or if there is incomplete virological suppression with cART

Laboratory tests play a key role in the diagnosis, monitoring and treatment of HIV infection (Table 3.1).

## The diagnosis of HIV infection

Tests to detect HIV antibody and screen for HIV infection were introduced in the mid-1980s. Over time, the screening tests have undergone refinement to improve diagnostic sensitivity in early infection and ensure recognition of genetically different HIV strains. Several confirmatory tests are also in routine use as part of the diagnostic algorithm. Thus, a combination of tests is needed to allow a specific and reliable diagnosis of HIV infection.

- *Screening tests* typically detect both HIV antibody and p24 antigen (fourth-generation assays) and are characterized by high sensitivity (low risk of false-negative results but a small risk of false-positive results).

- *Confirmatory tests* include additional fourth-generation tests using a different platform or format, and other antibody tests of typically lower sensitivity but high specificity (low risk of false-positive results).
- Whereas screening tests detect infection with HIV-1 (groups M and O) and HIV-2 without differentiating between the two, confirmatory tests also include assays that differentiate between HIV-1 and HIV-2.
- Confirmatory algorithms may include assays for the detection of p24 antigen alone in cases when recent infection is suspected, although HIV RNA (or less commonly proviral DNA) detection in peripheral blood provides an alternative approach.

**Table 3.1** Tests used to diagnose and monitor HIV infection.

| Test | Use | Notes |
|---|---|---|
| HIV antibodies | Diagnosis | Detected ~21–25 days after infection |
| | | Gold-standard assays detect antibodies against HIV-1 (groups M and O) and HIV-2 |
| | Staging | Certain assays identify the infection as recent (<−6 months) or established |
| p24 antigen | Diagnosis | Detected ~6 days earlier than antibodies |
| | | Combined HIV antibody/p24 antigen assays recommended as diagnostic standard |
| Plasma HIV-1 RNA load | Diagnosis | Detected ~9–11 days after infection |
| | | Can identify acute infection before HIV antibodies/p24 antigen become detectable |
| | Monitoring | In untreated patients, a nearly steady level ('set point') is observed within 6 months of infection, which predicts the rate of disease progression |
| | | Provides the key measure of successful response to cART |
| | | Provides a measure of HIV infectiousness |
| Proviral DNA | Diagnosis | Useful diagnostic test in for babies born to HIV + mothers. Also used in indeterminate or positive HIV serology with undetectable HIIV RNA in an untreated patient |
| | | No commercial assay |
| Drug resistance | Monitoring | Detection of resistance to antiretroviral drugs |
| HIV-1 tropism | Monitoring | Determines which co-receptor HIV-1 is likely to use and informs whether CCR5 antagonist effective treatment option |

*Source:* Table adapted from Asboe D, Aitken C, Boffito M, *et al.*, Reference 1.

*ABC of HIV and AIDS*, Sixth Edition. Edited by Michael W. Adler,
Simon G. Edwards, Robert F. Miller, Gulshan Sethi and Ian G. Williams.
© 2012 Blackwell Publishing Ltd. Published 2012 by Blackwell Publishing Ltd.

- HIV RNA or proviral DNA testing is also used to diagnose vertical HIV transmission in newborns from HIV-positive mothers as maternal HIV antibodies persist for up to 18 months, making serology results difficult to interpret. Children are typically tested at birth, 6 weeks and 12 weeks of age. A maternal sample is tested alongside the first infant sample to confirm that the assay can detect the maternal virus.

## The window period

Figure 3.1 illustrates the chronological order of detection of key serological and virological markers following HIV-1 infection. The time interval between HIV transmission and the ability to detect the infection in blood using serology tests is referred to as the 'window period'. This time period has considerably shortened with newer diagnostic tests (see below).

## Laboratory-based HIV screening tests

- First- and second-generation assays have now been discontinued.
- Third-generation assays are still part of many confirmatory algorithms. They are highly automated and employ recombinant viral proteins and synthetic peptides to detect HIV antibodies of the immunoglobulin (Ig)M, IgG and IgA classes.
- Fourth-generation assays, which allow the detection of both HIV antibodies and p24 antigen, are established as the standard of care for HIV screening in the UK. They have shortened the window period to typically 3–6 weeks of transmission. A negative test obtained 6 weeks after exposure excludes infection with a high degree of confidence, although a repeat test is recommended after 3 months for further reassurance, particularly in patients who have received post-exposure prophylaxis with cART.
- Non-specific (false-positive) reactivity has been occasionally observed following vaccinations, in patients with autoimmune diseases, in pregnant women, and in patients on dialysis or suffering from malignancies. Reactivity is usually weak and repeat testing of a follow-up sample is generally sufficient to exclude the infection.

Detection of HIV-1 RNA (or proviral DNA) in peripheral blood can further improve diagnostic sensitivity, and it is especially useful where screening tests give negative or equivocal results and a recent infection is strongly suspected.

Testing for proviral DNA in peripheral blood is recommended in cases where HIV-1 serology is indeterminate or positive but no HIV RNA is detected in plasma (Box 3.1).

---

Box 3.1 **Interpretation of HIV screening assays**

- Negative: unless within the window period after a possible exposure, the result is considered sufficient to exclude HIV infection
- Reactive: additional tests are required to confirm infection and differentiate between HIV-1 and HIV-2. A second blood sample is requested to confirm patient identity
- Equivocal/Indeterminate: this may reflect either non-specific reactivity or early infection. Management usually includes a battery of additional tests performed on the same sample, and if the results are still indeterminate, testing of a follow-up sample collected within 1 week of the first
- In cases where recent HIV infection is suspected and serology tests are negative or equivocal, HIV RNA (or proviral DNA) detection in peripheral blood is usually performed. A follow-up sample collected one week after the first sample is requested for repeat serology testing. In cases where HIV serology is positive (or equivocal) and no HIV RNA is detected in plasma, testing for proviral DNA is recommended

---

## Western blot and line immunoassay

Traditionally, HIV confirmatory tests have included western blot (WB), the line immunoassay (LIA), and the now rarely used radioimmunoprecipitation assay (RIPA). WB is expensive and labour intensive and in the UK is rarely used in routine diagnosis, being reserved for the investigation of samples with equivocal serology results. WB uses HIV-1 and HIV-2 denatured proteins blotted on a nitrocellulose membrane, which is cut into strips and probed with the patient's serum. HIV antibody is detected by an anti-human IgG antibody conjugated with an enzyme that, in the presence of substrate, will produce a coloured band. LIA uses a similar principle to WB but employs recombinant HIV antigens and synthetic peptides applied on nitrocellulose strips, which improves standardization and reduces background reactivity. The viral antigens include gp160, gp120, p66, p55, p51, gp41, p31, p24, p17 and p15, and established criteria are used for the interpretation of results.

## Rapid point-of-care HIV screening tests

Rapid, near-patient HIV screening tests have been developed in order to facilitate access to HIV testing, for example where laboratory infrastructure is limited, and to promote patient acceptability by facilitating and shortening the testing procedure. They are useful where a result can immediately influence management, for example in the assessment of the source of an exposure incident (e.g. needle-stick injury) or in untested pregnant women presenting during

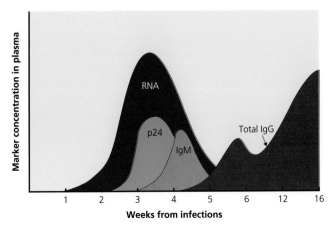

**Figure 3.1** Virological and serological markers during the first weeks after HIV-1 infection. Adapted from Murphy G, Parry JV. *Euro Surveill* 2008; 13(36) (www.eurosurveillance.org/ViewArticle.aspx?ArticleId=18966).

**Table 3.2** Point-of-care HIV antibody screening tests.

| Advantages | Disadvantages |
| --- | --- |
| Rapid, provide results <30 min | Expensive |
| Detect antibodies against HIV-1 (groups M and O) and HIV-2 | Reduced sensitivity in early infection compared with laboratory-based assays |
| Require simple equipment | Prone to operator errors |
| Easy to perform and interpret | Subjective interpretation of results |
| Avoid venopuncture | May give false positive results |
| Include a positive control | Reactive results require laboratory confirmation |
| Perform well compared with laboratory methods | Quality assurance complex to arrange |

Box 3.2 **Methodology of rapid point-of-care HIV screening based on immunochromatography**

- The test incorporates both antigen and signal reagent into a nitrocellulose strip. The sample added to an absorbent pad migrates through the strip and combines with a selenium colloid–antigen conjugate
- The mixture migrates through the solid phase to meet the immobilized HIV-1/2 recombinant antigens and synthetic peptides. Antibodies to HIV-1 and/or HIV-2 bind to the HIV antigens, forming a visible line at the patient window site
- If antibodies to HIV-1 and/or HIV-2 are absent, the mixture flows past the patient window without forming a line
- To ensure assay validity a procedural control line is applied to the strip beyond the HIV-antigen line

labour, in order to inform prophylactic measures. The tests typically employ capillary blood collected by fingerprick, are easy to perform by trained personnel and can provide a result in less than 30 minutes (Table 3.2).

The assays have good specificity and sensitivity in established HIV infection. Because of limitations in specificity, however, it is essential to obtain laboratory confirmation of all positive and indeterminate results. Studies have also indicated suboptimal sensitivity in recent infection relative to third- and fourth-generation laboratory screening tests. Rapid assays for the combined detection of HIV antibody and p24 antigen have recently been introduced that are expected to increase diagnostic sensitivity, although controlled data are currently limited.

Point-of-care test devices are also available for HIV antibody testing on saliva. The tests provide a good level of sensitivity for identification of established HIV infection where antibody levels are generally high. However, concerns have been raised regarding specificity of results.

The tests can be based on different immunodiagnostic principles. Those in common use are often based on the principle of immunochromatography (lateral flow) (Figure 3.2, Box 3.2)

## Serology tests to detect recent HIV-1 infection

Serology assays have been developed that can differentiate between HIV-1 infection acquired in the previous 4–6 months and established infection (Table 3.3). The different assays perform relatively well in population-based studies (e.g. to estimate HIV incidence) but are less reliable for individual patient management as their performance can be affected by factors such as disease stage, use of antiretroviral drugs, and possibly HIV-1 subtype.

## Virology tests for HIV detection and characterization

Virology tests for HIV detection and characterization include the quantification of HIV RNA in plasma ('viral load'), detection of antiretroviral drug resistance, and determination of HIV-1 tropism.

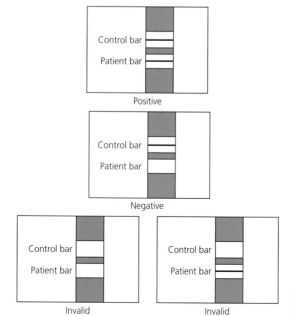

**Figure 3.2** Interpretation of results of rapid, point-of-care HIV screening tests.

**Table 3.3** Examples of assays for detecting recent HIV-1 infection.

| Assay | Principle |
|---|---|
| Detuned Assay with Abbott HIV 3A11 or Vironostika HIV-1 | High sensitivity/low sensitivity EIA. In early infection, a sample reactive in the sensitive test becomes nonreactive in the less-sensitive test. First test to be introduced but now discontinued. |
| BED-capture enzyme immune assay (CEIA) | Relative proportion of HIV IgG antibody and total IgG antibody present in a specific volume of serum. In early infection, the proportion of HIV-specific antibodies is lower than in established infection. Commercially available. |
| Avidity assay | In-house modifications of automated third generation HIV antibody tests (e.g. AxSYM or VITROS) that use sample pre-incubation with guanidine to disrupt low-affinity antibody/antigen interactions. In early infection, antibody/antigen bonds are easily disrupted leading to loss of reactivity compared with a sample incubated with control medium. |

**Table 3.4** Examples of commercial HIV-1 viral load assays and their range of quantification.

| Assay | Model | Quantification range (copies/mL) |
|---|---|---|
| Branched chain DNA (bDNA) | Bayer VERSANT HIV-1 RNA assay v. 3.0 | 50–500 000 |
| Reverse-transcription PCR (RT-PCR) | Roche Amplicor Monitor assay v. 1.5 | 400–750 000 (protocol 1) 50–75 000 (protocol 2) |
| Nucleic acid sequence based amplification (NASBA) + real-time molecular beacon detection | BioMerieux NucliSens EasyQ assay | 50–3 000 000 |
| Real-time RT PCR | Roche COBASR TaqManR HIV-1 v.2 assay | 20–10 000 000 |
| | Abbott RealTime HIV-1 assay | 40–10 000 000 |
| Reverse transcriptase activity measured in ELISA | Cavidi ExaVir Load v.3 assay | ~200–600 000 |

## Viral load

The HIV-1 RNA load in plasma is a marker of infectiousness and a potent predictor of the rate of CD4 decline, disease progression and mortality. In patients on combination antiretroviral therapy (cART), the viral load provides the main surrogate marker for the clinical efficacy of cART. Following initiation of cART, a rapid decline in viral load is seen in the first few days followed by a slower decline that brings the level below 50 copies/mL within 16–24 weeks. Clinical trials and observational studies indicate that achieving and maintain a viral load below 50 copies/mL predicts long-term viral load suppression and immunological and clinical benefit.

Commercial assays show excellent correlation and reliably detect and quantify all major HIV-1 group M subtypes and circulating recombinant forms (CRFs). Some assays also detect group O viruses, but no commercial assay is available for the quantification of group N or group P HIV-1 strains, or for HIV-2 (Table 3.4).

Molecular viral load assays in routine use in high-income countries require expensive instruments and reagents, sophisticated laboratory facilities to minimize the risk of contamination, regular and stable electricity supply and highly skilled laboratory technicians who are proficient in molecular biology techniques. These factors have to date limited their implementation in resource-limited settings. Highly portable viral load assays suitable for settings with a limited laboratory infrastructure are currently being developed.

Viral load assays were introduced in routine clinical practice in the 1990s. Over time they have undergone refinement to improve the sensitivity of detection and performance with genetically diverging HIV strains. Mismatches between primers and probes and RNA target sequences, due to HIV genetic variations, can still result in falsely low or undetectable viral loads in some samples. Testing with a second method is recommended when the viral load results are not consistent with the patient's history.

## HIV proviral DNA testing

Proviral DNA testing is mainly used in two scenarios: for confirmation of diagnosis in certain adults where results of screening and confirmatory tests are inconclusive or where a positive serology in an untreated patient is accompanied by undetectable HIV RNA (although a negative result does not exclude infection), and for the diagnosis of infants born to HIV-infected women.

## Antiretroviral drug resistance

HIV strains resistant to antiretroviral drugs carry key mutations in the targets of cART. The mutants are generated spontaneously during virus replication because of the high error rate and lack of proofreading activity of the viral reverse transcriptase enzyme, which transcribes the HIV genome. Incomplete suppression of virus replication during cART leads to their emergence and evolution (Figure 3.3). Drug-resistant mutants may also be transmitted. Among newly diagnosed patients in the UK and Western Europe, approximately 7–10% have evidence of transmitted drug resistance (Box 3.3).

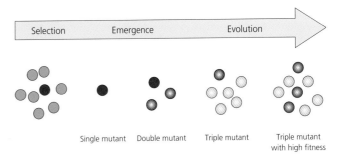

**Figure 3.3** Selection, emergence and evolution of drug-resistant mutants during virus replication in the presence of drug pressure.

---

Box 3.3 **Principles of antiretroviral drug resistance**

Resistant mutants before therapy is introduced

- are generated spontaneously during virus replication
- usually display reduced ability to replicate ('viral fitness')
- are present at low frequency within the virus population

Resistant mutants during therapy

- acquire a selective advantage over drug susceptible virus
- are selected by drug pressure if virus suppression is incomplete
- with ongoing virus replication become dominant within the virus population
- continue to evolve under drug pressure with increasing levels of resistance
- over time acquire mutations that compensate for reduced fitness

Resistant mutants after therapy is discontinued

- lose the replication advantage
- are outgrown by drug-susceptible virus
- persist at low frequency in circulating virus and are archived in latently infected cells
- can re-emerge rapidly when drug pressure is reintroduced

There are two main approaches for detecting drug resistance in routine practice: genotypic and phenotypic testing. Both methods typically use viral RNA recovered from the patient's plasma.

- In phenotypic testing, the viral genomic regions are transfected into a laboratory vector generating a recombinant virus that can be grown *in vitro* in the presence of escalating drug concentration.
- In genotypic testing, which is more commonly used in the UK and the rest of Europe, drug resistance mutations in the viral genomic region of interest are detected by automated population sequencing. Current targets include the viral protease, reverse transcriptase and integrase enzymes and the gp41 envelope protein. The sequence is compared with a reference sequence and changes in key amino acids at positions that are known to confer a resistant phenotype are reported. Several interpretation systems are available freely online to aid the interpretation of genotypic resistance profiles (e.g. Stanford University HIV Resistance Database).
- The assays cannot detect resistant variants present at low frequency (<20–30%) within the virus population. Therefore during treatment failure, a resistance test should be performed

while the patient is still receiving therapy to ensure optimal performance, as resistant mutants decay below the assay detection threshold after therapy is discontinued. Transmitted drug-resistant mutants show different kinetics as many they decay slowly and remain detectable for years after infection in the absence of drug pressure. New assays are currently under development that improve the sensitivity of detection (e.g., ultra-deep sequencing).

## HIV-1 tropism

CCR5 and CXCR4 are the major cellular co-receptors involved in HIV-1 entry into the host target cells. According to the ability of the virus to use one or the other co-receptor, HIV-1 variants are classified as R5, X4 or R5/X4 dual tropic if using both co-receptors. Throughout infection, the detection of only R5 virus in plasma is most common. CXCR4-using variants are more likely to be detected as mixed populations of R5 and X4 strains in patients with advanced disease. The detection of exclusively X4 virus in clinical samples is uncommon.

CCR5 antagonists such as maraviroc have been recently developed for the treatment of HIV-1 infection. Since their activity is specific for R5 tropic virus, a test to determine HIV-1 tropism is required prior to use. Genotypic tropism testing methods have been developed based on the principle that the V3 loop of the envelope gp120 glycoprotein is the major determinant of co-receptor usage.

## Further reading

Asboe D, Aitken C, Boffito M, *et al.* British HIV Association guidelines for the routine investigation and monitoring of adult HIV-1-infected individuals 2011. HIV Med 2012;13:1–44.

Geretti AM. HIV testing and monitoring. *Medicine* 2009;37:326–329.

Murphy G, Parry JV. Assays for the detection of recent infection with human immunodeficiency virus type 1. *Eurosurveillance* 2008;13(36).

Pillay D, Geretti AM, Weiss RA. Human Immunodeficiency viruses. In Zuckerman AJ, Banatvala JE, Griffiths PD, *et al.* (eds) *Principles and Practise of Clinical Virology*, 6th edition. Wiley-Blackwell, 2009;38:897–938.

Vandamme AM, Camacho RJ, Ceccherini-Silberstein F, *et al.* European recommendations for the clinical use of HIV drug resistance testing: 2011 update. *AIDS Rev* 2011;13:77–108.

Vandekerckhove LP, Wensing AM, Kaiser R, *et al.* European guidelines on the clinical management of HIV-1 tropism testing. *Lancet Infect Dis* 2011;11:394–407.

## CHAPTER 4

# HIV Testing: Strategies to Prevent Late Diagnosis

*A. Palfreeman[1] and E. Fox[2]*

[1]University Hospitals of Leicester, Leicester, UK
[2]Kent and Canterbury Hospital, Canterbury, UK

---

**OVERVIEW**

- HIV is now a treatable medical condition, and the majority of those living with the virus remain fit and well on treatment
- Approximately a quarter of all HIV positive individuals in the UK and USA are unaware of their diagnosis
- More widespread HIV testing is recommended to prevent late diagnosis and onward transmission
- National guidelines on HIV testing were published in 2008 (UK)
- Many urban areas in the UK have an HIV prevalence greater than that recommended for screening (2/1000)
- Availability of point of care HIV tests may help to increase uptake of HIV testing
- HIV testing should be normalized. All doctors, nurses and midwives should be able to obtain informed consent for an HIV test in the same way that they currently do for any other medical investigation

---

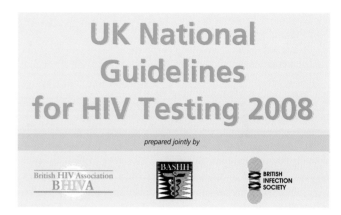

**Figure 4.1** UK National Guidelines for HIV Testing 2008.

## Introduction

There has been a significant change in national and international guidance for HIV testing since earlier editions of this book. In 2006, the US Centers for Disease Control and Prevention (CDC) issued expanded recommendations for HIV in the USA. In the UK, national guidelines on HIV testing were developed in 2008 (Figure 4.1). These were endorsed by NICE guidance and a Parliamentary select committee on HIV and AIDS in 2011.

In the past, most HIV testing took place within Genito-Urinary Medicine clinics, with an emphasis placed on pre-test counselling to ensure that valid consent was obtained. This was appropriate in the earlier years of the HIV epidemic when HIV was rare and untreatable, with HIV-positive individuals facing widespread stigma and discrimination. However, HIV has now become a chronic treatable condition, and late diagnosis of HIV infection is now the most important factor associated with HIV-related morbidity and mortality in the UK.

Around a quarter of all HIV-positive individuals remain undiagnosed in the UK, and an estimated 30% of individuals are diagnosed very late (CD4 count <200 cells/μL). Late diagnosis is more prevalent in older age groups, heterosexual men and black and ethnic minority populations. Many of these patients have missed opportunities for earlier diagnosis in that studies have shown that a significant proportion have been seen for care by their general practitioners or other physicians with HIV-related symptoms but the diagnosis of HIV was overlooked. In addition to risks to their own health, undiagnosed individuals run the risk of unwittingly transmitting their infection to others and so fuelling the HIV epidemic.

The 2008 National Guidelines on HIV testing aim to reduce the proportion of HIV-positive individuals unaware of their infection. The guidelines recommend that HIV testing should be normalized to become a routine medical investigation carried out in many medical settings, and that obtaining consent for an HIV test should be within the competence of any healthcare professional.

In 2011 NICE issued separate guidelines on HIV testing aimed at black African communities and guidance aimed at men who have sex with other men. These recommend increased offers of testing in these populations, as both these communities bear a disproportionate burden of HIV disease.

## Who to test for HIV

It is now recommended that an HIV test is offered on an opt-out basis to all patients presenting for care:

*ABC of HIV and AIDS*, Sixth Edition. Edited by Michael W. Adler,
Simon G. Edwards, Robert F. Miller, Gulshan Sethi and Ian G. Williams.
© 2012 Blackwell Publishing Ltd. Published 2012 by Blackwell Publishing Ltd.

- in a number of specific settings
- who are members of specific higher risk groups
- who have certain medical conditions.

An opt-out test ensures that the test becomes a part of the routine standard of care while still allowing patients the right to decline a test.

The settings where an HIV test should be routine are those where patients are at increased risk of HIV infection, or, in the case of antenatal services, where it is important not to miss the diagnosis to prevent onward transmission to the baby (Box 4.1).

---

**Box 4.1  Specific settings where HIV testing should be routine**

- GUM/sexual health clinics
- Antenatal services
- Termination of pregnancy services
- Drug dependency programmes
- Healthcare services for those diagnosed with tuberculosis, hepatitis B, hepatitis C and lymphoma

---

HIV testing has been routinely offered to all patients attending sexually transmitted infection (STI) clinics since 1999, with uptake of over 70%, and in antenatal clinics since 2001 with uptake of over 90%. Women undergoing termination of pregnancy have a prevalence of HIV of up to 1%. High numbers of patients attending drug dependency programmes will have injected drugs. Over 5% of patients with tuberculosis (TB) in England and Wales are HIV positive and TB is often the first AIDS-defining condition. Lymphoma is much more common in HIV infection than in the general population. Hepatitis B and C, like HIV, are blood-borne viruses and many individuals are dually infected.

Routine HIV testing should also be offered to all patients presenting to acute medicine or registering in primary care in parts of the country where the local HIV prevalence is greater than two per 1000 among 15–59 year olds. Routine screening at this prevalence or higher is known to be cost-effective. The Health Protection Agency produces data that maps HIV prevalence by area (Figure 4.2).

Around a fifth of the population in England live in a high prevalence area, the majority of them in London. Published data from both the USA and the UK have shown that the routine offer of an HIV test in a variety of settings (which have historically been thought to be difficult to roll out HIV testing) have been shown to be cost-effective, acceptable to patients and effective in identifying previously undiagnosed individuals.

The groups of people who should be offered a routine HIV test are those known to be at increased risk of HIV infection (Box 4.2).

---

**Box 4.2  Groups of people who should be offered a routine HIV test**

1 Patients where HIV enters the differential diagnosis
2 Patients diagnosed with a sexually transmitted infection
3 Sexual partners of individuals known to be HIV positive
4 Men who have had sexual contact with other men
5 Female sexual contacts of men who have sex with men
6 Individuals who have ever injected drugs
7 Men and women from countries of high HIV prevalence (>1%)
8 Men and women who have had sexual contact abroad or in the UK with individuals from countries of high HIV prevalence
9 The following groups in accordance with existing guidelines

   – blood donors
   – dialysis patients
   – organ transplant donors and recipients

---

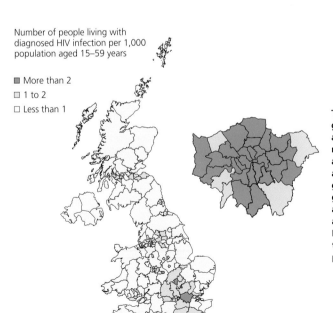

Number of people living with diagnosed HIV infection per 1,000 population aged 15–59 years

■ More than 2
□ 1 to 2
□ Less than 1

**The UK national guidelines for testing advocate the offer and recommendation to accept an HIV test to all adults registering in general practice and general medical admissions patients in areas where diagnosed HIV prevalence is greater than 2 per 1,000 population.**

**Figure 4.2** Prevalence of diagnosed HIV Infection, UK, 2009. *Source:* Annual survey of HIV-infected persons accessing care. Reproduced with permission of the Health Protection Agency.

**Table 4.1** HIV clinical indicator conditions.

| | AIDS-defining conditions | Other conditions where HIV testing should be recommended |
|---|---|---|
| Respiratory | Tuberculosis<br>Pneumocystis | Bacterial pneumonia<br>Aspergillosis |
| Neurology | Cerebral toxoplasmosis<br>Primary cerebral lymphoma<br>Cryptococcal meningitis<br>Progressive multifocal leucoencephalopathy | Aseptic meningitis/encephalitis cerebral abscess<br>Space occupying lesion of unknown cause<br>Guillain–Barré syndrome<br>Transverse myelitis<br>Peripheral neuropathy<br>Dementia<br>Leucoencephalopathy |
| Dermatology | Kaposi sarcoma | Severe or recalcitrant seborrhoeic dermatitis<br>Severe or recalcitrant psoriasis, multidermatomal or recurrent herpes zoster |
| Gastroenterology | Persistent cryptosporidiosis | Oral candidiasis<br>Oral hairy leucoplakia<br>Chronic diarrhoea of unknown cause<br>Weight loss of unknown cause, salmonella, shigella or campylobacter, hepatitis B infection<br>Hepatitis C infection |
| Oncology | Non-Hodgkin's lymphoma | Anal cancer or anal intraepithelial dysplasia<br>Lung cancer<br>Seminoma<br>Head and neck cancer<br>Hodgkin's lymphoma<br>Castleman's disease |
| Gynaecology | Cervical cancer | Vaginal intraepithelial neoplasia<br>Cervical intraepithelial neoplasia Grade 2 or above |
| Haematology | | Any unexplained blood dyscrasia including:<br>• neutropenia<br>• thrombocytopenia<br>• lymphopenia |
| Ophthalmology | Cytomegalovirus retinitis | Infective retinal diseases including herpesviruses and toxoplasma<br>Any unexplained retinopathy |
| ENT | | Lymphadenopathy of unknown cause<br>Chronic parotitis<br>Lymphoepithelial parotid cysts |
| Other | | Pyrexia of unknown origin<br>Any lymphadenopathy of unknown cause<br>Mononucleosis-like syndrome (primary HIV infection)<br>Any sexually transmitted infection |

The clinical indicator conditions, where HIV enters the differential diagnosis, which should prompt a routine offer of an HIV test, are listed in Table 4.1.

## Frequency of HIV testing

Most of the time a single negative test is sufficient to rule out the diagnosis of HIV. A repeat test may be necessary if testing for HIV occurred within the window period (see Chapter 3).

Certain groups of patients should be tested more frequently:

- Men who have sex with men–test at least annually, or more frequently if they have symptoms suggestive of HIV seroconversion illness or high-risk behaviour.
- Injecting drug users – test annually or more frequently if they have symptoms suggestive of seroconversion illness.

- Pregnant women – if at ongoing high risk (or become unwell with seroconversion-like symptoms during pregnancy) repeat a test at 34–36 weeks. A repeat test should also be offered to women who have refused an HIV test earlier in pregnancy.

## Which test to use

Testing for HIV may be performed on laboratory-based blood tests or via rapid point of care tests (see Chapter 3). Rapid tests are becoming increasingly used as they are acceptable to patients and can overcome logistical issues in increasing HIV testing uptake in some settings. They rely on either serum from fingerprick or saliva from a mouth swab and can give the patient a result in a few minutes (Figure 4.3).

Occasionally an HIV test is inconclusive or gives an equivocal result and a laboratory-based blood test is required.

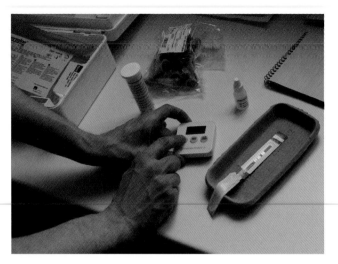

**Figure 4.3** Rapid HIV test.

## Pre-test discussion (Box 4.3)

Consent should be obtained prior to an HIV test, as with any planned investigation. Advising the patient that a routine HIV test is recommended and the reasons why it is recommended, then asking for permission to do the test while giving the patient time to ask questions, is the most appropriate way of gaining consent. If a patient refuses a test, the reasons for this should be explored to ensure that they do not hold incorrect beliefs about the virus or the consequences of testing. For example, some individuals believe that having a routine HIV test affects future life insurance; this is no longer correct following the 1994 Association of British Insurers (ABI) Code of Practice (Figure 4.4).

---

Box 4.3 **HIV pre-test discussion**

As a minimum the pre-test discussion should cover

- the benefits of testing to the individual
- details of how the result will be given

---

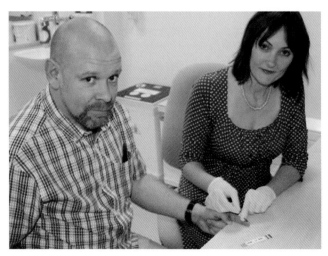

**Figure 4.4** Performing an HIV test after HIV pre-test discussion.

Written consent is not necessary, but the offer of an HIV test should be documented in the patient's notes together with any relevant discussion that has taken place. If the patient refuses a test, the reasons for this should be recorded.

Some groups of patients may need additional help to make a decision, for example children and young people, those with learning difficulties or mental health problems, and those for whom English is not their first language. It is essential to take time to ensure that these patients have understood what is proposed, and why.

For young children in whom testing is indicated, there may be issues about parental acceptance of the need to test and a possible positive diagnosis. This is a complex area, but the overriding consideration is the best interests of the child, and multidisciplinary decision-making and expert advice should be sought where appropriate, including legal advice.

## Giving HIV test results

Arrangements on when and how the result will be received by the patient should be agreed at the time of testing. For the majority of individuals, if the result is not thought likely to be positive there is no need to deliver the result face to face.

Face-to-face provision of HIV test results is strongly encouraged for the following:

- ward-based patients;
- patients more likely to have an HIV positive result;
- those with mental health problems/suicide risk;
- those for whom English is a second language;
- young people under 16 years;
- highly anxious or vulnerable individuals.

### Post-test discussion for individuals who are negative

These individuals should be offered screening for sexually transmitted infections and advice around risk reduction and behaviour change, including discussion relating to HIV post-exposure prophylaxis (PEP) if at higher risk of repeat exposure to HIV infection. This is best achieved by onward referral to GUM/HIV services or voluntary sector agencies.

If the individual is still within the window period after a specific exposure (<12 weeks), the need for a repeat HIV test should be discussed.

### Post-test discussion for individuals who test HIV positive

Prior to giving a positive result, it is essential to have established a clear pathway for onward referral to the HIV specialist team.

The result of a positive HIV test should be given in a confidential environment face to face with the patient by the testing clinician or team (Box 4.4). A result should not be given to any third party, including relatives or other clinical teams, unless the patient has specifically agreed to this. This is in line with the general principles of confidentiality for any medical condition as laid down by the General Medical Council.

Box 4.4 **Giving a positive HIV result**

A positive HIV result should be given

- by the team/clinician who consented the patient
- face to face
- in a confidential environment
- using clear language

If a patient's first language is not English, it is considered good practice to use a translation service rather than family member for purposes of confidentiality. Establish that the patient understands what a positive and a negative result mean in terms of infection with HIV, as some patients interpret 'positive' as good news.

The HIV team should then see the patient as soon as possible to assess disease stage, consider the need for treatment and carry out partner notification (see Chapter 6).

## Summary

The advent of effective treatment has transformed HIV infection into a chronic manageable disease with a near-normal lifespan. However, approximately one-quarter of individuals are unaware of their infection and are diagnosed late, with significant impact on individual and public health. Increasing the routine offer of HIV testing, normalizing the testing process, and improved recognition of clinical indicator diseases by hospital clinicians should significantly improve the current situation. All doctors, nurses and midwives should be able to obtain informed consent for an HIV test.

## Further reading

BHIVA. Time to test for HIV: Expanded healthcare and community HIV testing in England. (www.bhiva.org/documents/Conferences/TimeToTest2010/Time_to_test_for_HIV_Interim_report_Dec_2010.pdf).

British HIV Association, British Association for Sexual Health and HIV, British Infection Society. UK. National Guidelines for HIV Testing 2008. (www.bhiva.org/documents/Guidelines/Testing/GlinesHIVTest08.pdf. Sept 2008).

MMWR. Revised Recommendations for HIV Testing of Adults, Adolescents, and Pregnant Women in Health-Care Settings. September 22, 2006/55 (RR14);1–17. (www.cdc.gov/mmwr/preview/mmwrhtml/rr5514a1.htm).

National Institute for Health and Clinical Excellence. Increasing the uptake of HIV testing to reduce undiagnosed infection and prevent transmission among black African communities living in England. National Institute for Health and Clinical Excellence public health guidance 33, March 2011. (www.nice.org.uk/PH33).

National Institute for Health and Clinical Excellence. Increasing the uptake of HIV testing to reduce undiagnosed infection and prevent transmission among men who have sex with men. National Institute for Health and Clinical Excellence public health guidance 34, March 2011. (www.nice.org.uk/PH34).

Select Committee on HIV and AIDs in the United Kingdom – First Report No vaccine, no cure: HIV and AIDS in the United Kingdom. September 2011. (www.publications.parliament.uk/pa/ld201012/ldselect/ldaids/188/18802.htm).

# CHAPTER 5

# Clinical Staging and Natural History of Untreated HIV Infection

M. Tenant-Flowers[1] and A. Mindel[2]

[1]King's College Hospital, London, UK
[2]Westmead Hospital, Westmead, Sydney, NSW, Australia

**OVERVIEW**

- HIV infection causes a spectrum of disease
- The Centers for Disease Control in the USA developed the most widely used classification for HIV disease based on clinical symptoms and signs, the presence of certain conditions and the degree of immunosuppression as measured by the CD4 lymphocyte count
- Untreated HIV infection leads to an inexorable decline in CD4 cell counts leading to immunosuppression and opportunistic infections
- Factors influencing disease progression include older age, higher plasma viral loads and severely symptomatic primary HIV infection

## Introduction

Infection with HIV causes a spectrum of disease ranging from primary HIV infection (PHI) in the very early stage of infection to, in the absence of cART, diseases associated with immune suppression and eventually death. Between PHI and the development of AIDS there is a progressive loss of CD4 lymphocytes with the patient's CD4 falling by between 50 and 100 cells/μL per year. Individuals are often asymptomatic during this phase. The median time from infection to developing AIDS in untreated people is 10 years (range 18 months to 25 years). The rate of progression can vary significantly, with some individuals progressing to AIDS within a couple of years ('rapid progressors') and others maintaining a good immune system more than 10 years later ('slow progressors'). Higher plasma HIV viral loads and severe symptomatic PHI are associated with faster progression to AIDS. Less than 1% of patients will be able to control HIV viraemia without combination antiretroviral therapy (cART) and these patients rarely develop immune suppression or AIDS. These individuals are known as 'elite controllers'. Some children with vertically transmitted HIV are surviving with asymptomatic infection for more than 20 years.

Prior to the availability of antiretrovirals, the mean survival time after an diagnosis of AIDS was less than 2 years. The introduction of

cART has revolutionized prognosis and when commenced early in HIV infection the life expectancy with HIV infection may approach normal.

The Centers for Disease Control (CDC) in the USA developed the most widely used classification for HIV disease based on clinical symptoms and signs, the presence of certain conditions and the degree of immunosuppression as measured by the CD4 lymphocyte count. This was updated by the CDC in 1993 to classify all HIV-infected persons with CD4 lymphocyte counts of <200 cells/μL as fulfilling the AIDS-defining illness criteria (Boxes 5.1–5.3). The

---

Box 5.1 **Conditions included in the 1993 AIDS surveillance case definition**

- Candidiasis of bronchi, trachea or lungs
- Candidiasis, oesophageal
- Cervical cancer, invasive
- Coccidioidomycosis, disseminated or extrapulmonary
- Cryptococcosis, extrapulmonary
- Cryptosporidiosis, chronic intestinal (greater than 1 month's duration)
- Cytomegalovirus disease (other than liver, spleen, or nodes)
- Cytomegalovirus retinitis (with loss of vision)
- Encephalopathy, HIV related
- Herpes simplex: chronic ulcer(s) (greater than 1 month's duration); or bronchitis, pneumonitis or oesophagitis
- Histoplasmosis, disseminated or extrapulmonary
- Isosporiasis, chronic intestinal (greater than 1 month's duration)
- Kaposi sarcoma
- Lymphoma, Burkitt's (or equivalent term)
- Lymphoma, immunoblastic (or equivalent term)
- Lymphoma, primary, of brain
- *Mycobacterium avium* complex or *M. kansasii*, disseminated or extrapulmonary
- *Mycobacterium tuberculosis*, any site (pulmonary or extrapulmonary)
- Mycobacterium, other species or unidentified species, disseminated or extrapulmonary
- Pneumocystis jirovecii pneumonia
- Pneumonia, recurrent
- Progressive multifocal leucoencephalopathy
- Salmonella septicemia, recurrent
- Toxoplasmosis of brain
- Wasting syndrome due to HIV

---

*ABC of HIV and AIDS*, Sixth Edition. Edited by Michael W. Adler, Simon G. Edwards, Robert F. Miller, Gulshan Sethi and Ian G. Williams.
© 2012 Blackwell Publishing Ltd. Published 2012 by Blackwell Publishing Ltd.

classification of the stage of HIV infection provides a framework for categorizing morbidity and immunosuppression and is an important tool for HIV surveillance. Prior to the widespread availability of cART (which has the ability to restore HIV-induced immune suppression) it was very important as it helped to estimate an individual's prognosis and to make decisions about when to start opportunistic infection prophylaxis and available cART.

---

Box 5.2 **Clinical categories of HIV infection**

**Category A**

This consists of one or more of the conditions listed below in

- Asymptomatic HIV infection
- Persistent generalized lymphadenopathy
- Acute (primary) HIV infection with accompanying illness or history of acute HIV infection

**Category B**

This consists of symptomatic conditions

- Bacillary angiomatosis
- Candidiasis, oropharyngeal (thrush)
- Candidiasis, vulvovaginal; persistent, frequent, or poorly responsive to therapy
- Cervical dysplasia (moderate or severe)/cervical carcinoma in situ
- Constitutional symptoms, such as fever (38.5°C) or diarrhoea lasting greater than 1 month
- Hairy leucoplakia, oral
- Herpes zoster (shingles), involving at least two distinct episodes or more than one dermatome
- Idiopathic thrombocytopenic purpura
- Listeriosis
- Pelvic inflammatory disease, particularly if complicated by tubo-ovarian abscess
- Peripheral neuropathy

**Category C**

This includes the clinical conditions listed in the AIDS surveillance case definition (see Box 5.1)

---

Box 5.3 **CD4+ T-lymphocyte count criteria included in the 1993 AIDS surveillance case definition**

All HIV-infected persons who have less than 200 CD4+ T-lymphocytes/uL, or a CD4+ T-lymphocyte percentage of total lymphocytes of less than 14.

---

## Primary HIV infection (PHI)

PHI is the time between initial infection to the development of antibodies against HIV. During this period the individual frequently develops symptoms compatible with an acute viral infection. This is also known as 'HIV seroconversion illness'.

The clinical presentation ranges from a mild glandular fever-like illness with a rash to an encephalopathy. Common symptoms and

signs are shown in Box 5.4. Severe symptoms are rare. The onset of PHI symptoms within 3 weeks, symptoms that last for longer than 2 weeks and central nervous system involvement are associated with rapid progression to AIDS. The differential diagnosis of a mild seroconversion illness is protean and, without a high index of suspicion and a history indicating relevant risk behaviours or factors, the diagnosis may be missed. It is particularly important to exclude secondary syphilis.

---

Box 5.4 **Clinical manifestations of primary HIV infection**

- 96% fever
- 74% lymphadenopathy
- 70% pharyngitis
- 70% rash*
- 54% myalgia
- 32% diarrhoea
- 32% headache
- 27% nausea and vomiting
- 14% hepatosplenomegaly
- 13% weight loss
- 12% oral candida
- 12% neurological symptoms

*Erythematous, maculopapular rash mainly on face and trunk with or without mucocutaneous ulcers of mouth, oesophagus or genitals.

---

The appropriate diagnostic tests for PHI that should be carried out on serial blood samples include tests for HIV antibodies and antigen. All laboratories in the UK should now be using a fourth-generation combined antibody/antigen test which should detect primary infection, i.e. within the first few weeks (Chapter 3).

At the time of PHI there is sometimes a high rate of viral replication, leading to a transient rise in HIV viral load with concomitant immunosuppression due to a short-lived (occasionally dramatic) fall in the CD4 count (Figure 5.1).

Rarely, this may result in manifestations of HIV disease normally seen later in the disease, e.g. oral candida (Figure 5.2) leading to occasional diagnostic confusion as to the stage of HIV infection.

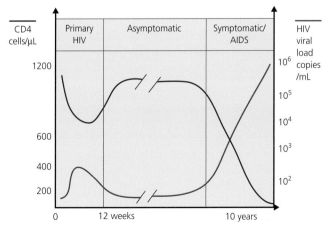

**Figure 5.1** Association between virological, immunological and clinical events and time course of HIV infection.

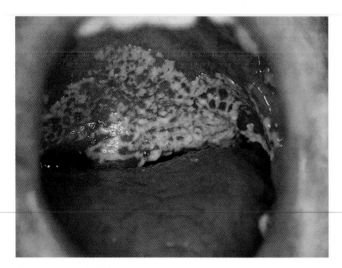

**Figure 5.2** Oral candida.

Sometimes, this can be resolved by taking a full sexual history to establish when HIV might have been transmitted. Newer virological assays should also be used to identify HIV seroconversion (see Chapter 3) together with serial viral load and CD4 cell assays. Over time, after PHI, the viral load will fall and the CD4 count rise. During PHI initiation of cART is usually only considered in the presence of severe symptoms (especially central nervous system involvement), an AIDS-defining diagnosis or severe immunosuppression (CD4 < 350 cells/μL).

There is considerable interest into the efficacy of cART during PHI to decrease long-term damage to the immune system, delay disease progression and prevent transmission (see Chapter 19). It is postulated that HIV may be more susceptible during PHI to cART due to the relatively low diversity of replicating virus particles, the reduced ability of the predominantly non-syncytium-inducing (NSI) strains of virus to infect a wide variety of cell types and the enhanced immune response seen at this time. However, if not started early in the course of PHI (i.e. within 6 months) the theoretical advantage may be lost and, in any case, has to be balanced against an uncertain outcome, drug toxicity, adherence difficulties and the possibility of developing resistant virus and limiting future treatment options.

Individuals with PHI are usually extremely infectious at this stage due to very high levels of HIV within the body; therefore, contacts need to be carefully screened and followed up, PEP offered if appropriate and advice given to avoid onward transmission.

## Asymptomatic infection

After PHI, HIV antibodies continue to be detectable in the blood. The amount of virus in blood and lymphoid tissues falls to significantly lower levels than seen in PHI and the rate of HIV replication slows, although it does not cease. CD4 counts are generally above 350 cells/μL. This phase may persist for 15 years or more (Figure 5.1). The role of cART during asymptomatic infection is discussed in Chapter 19.

Transmission is still possible despite the viral load being lower than PHI and, as the progression rate to AIDS varies widely, monitoring should continue to ensure that cART is offered at the optimum time.

## Persistent generalised lymphadenopathy

This is defined as lymphadenopathy that persists for at least 3 months, in at least two extra-inguinal sites and is not due to any other cause. The differential diagnosis of lymphadenopathy in HIV is wide and includes *Mycobacterium* TB and lymphoma. Mediastinal and intra-abdominal lymphadenopathy are not part of this syndrome and require further investigation to exclude infection and neoplasia. The presence of persistent generalized lymphadenopathy does not affect disease progression. This alone is not an indication to start HIV treatment.

## Symptomatic HIV infection before the development of AIDS

The progression of HIV infection results in a decline in immune competence that occurs due to the increased replication of HIV from sites where it has been latent. The exact triggers for this reactivation are still poorly understood. As the disease progresses, infected persons may suffer from constitutional symptoms, skin and mouth problems (see Figures 5.2–5.5 and Chapter 14) and haematological disorders, many of which are easy to treat and alleviate. A decrease in HIV viral load in response to the introduction of cART often corresponds to a complete or partial resolution of these symptoms.

## Constitutional symptoms

Common constitutional symptoms associated with symptomatic HIV infection include malaise, fevers, night sweats, weight loss and diarrhoea. The exact criteria for diagnosing the AIDS-defining HIV wasting syndrome are the combination of 10% weight loss from

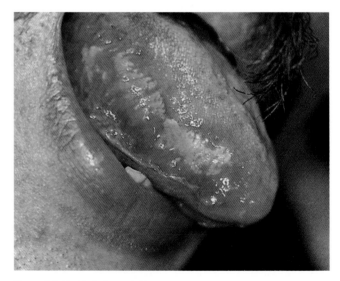

**Figure 5.3** Oral hairy leucoplakia.

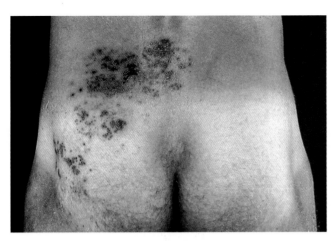

**Figure 5.4** Unidermatomal shingles caused by varicella zoster.

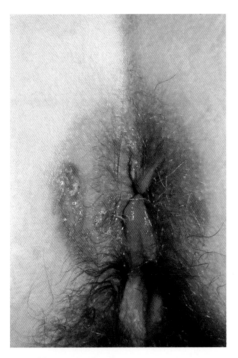

**Figure 5.5** Perianal herpes simplex virus.

baseline and one of fever or diarrhoea lasting at least 1 month. Many patients find these symptoms worrying and debilitating and they should always be investigated to diagnose treatable causes other than HIV.

## HIV and haematological problems

Haematological abnormalities are common in HIV disease and usually have no adverse effect. These include lymphopenia, moderate neutropenia (which may be linked to ethnicity), a normochromic, normocytic anaemia and thrombocytopenia. Bone marrow biopsies usually indicate trilineage dysplasia and are not routinely indicated in the absence of coexisting fever, diarrhoea or lymphadenopathy, which may indicate mycobacterial infection or neoplasia. Many

of these abnormalities wholly or partially resolve after cART is initiated.

## Non-AIDS diagnoses for which cART has treatment benefit irrespective of CD4 count

The defining features of AIDS are the 'persistent and profound selective decrease in the function as well as number of T lymphocytes of the helper/inducer subset and a possible activation of the suppressor/cytotoxic subset'. However, alongside this immunosuppression an immune dysregulation occurs which affects natural killer cells, plasmacytoid dendritic cells and CD8 T-cell function. Owing to this complex immunological interplay, HIV-related disease processes can still occur at 'high CD4 counts' and so the clinical course of patients with these conditions will benefit from the initiation of cART in order to optimise immune control.

Examples include:

- idiopathic thrombocytopenic purpura (ITP)
- thrombotic thrombocytopenic purpura (TTP)
- HIV-associated nephropathy (HIVAN)
- severe refractory psoriasis
- pulmonary arterial hypertension
- HIV vasculitis

## Risk of progression and the value of surrogate markers

Predicting how soon a patient will progress to symptomatic disease or AIDS is an issue with which physicians continue to grapple. Variables associated with rapid disease progression and some host and viral factors which appear to be protective are shown in Box 5.5.

---

Box 5.5 **Factors affecting HIV disease progression**

**Factors which increase the rate of progression**
- Older age
- PHI – early onset <3 weeks and prolonged symptoms >2 weeks
- Higher HIV viral load
- Baseline albumin <35 mg/mL
- CXCR4 (syncitium inducing) strain of HIV
- Rapid rate of fall of absolute CD4 cell count
- Route of infection – blood transfusion

**Factors which appear protective**
- CCR5 co-receptor delta 32 mutation
- Certain HLA mutations
- Vpr mutation of HIV viral protein

---

Many laboratory indices have been used as prognostic indicators, both to evaluate disease progression and treatment efficacy. The most widely used are the CD4 absolute lymphocyte count or percentage and the HIV viral load. At least two CD4 measurements

**Table 5.1** Association between major clinical events in HIV infection and CD4 cell count – potential indications for prophylaxis.

| CD4 cell count (cells/μL) | Clinical event |
|---|---|
| <200 | Pneumocystis pneumonia |
| <100 | Toxoplasmosis |
| | Cryptococcosis |
| | Candidal oesophagitis |
| <50 | Disseminated cytomegalovirus |
| | Disseminated *Mycobacterium avium* complex |

should be obtained before initiating prophylaxis for opportunistic infections or cART as the CD4 count is subject to diurnal and seasonal variation and reduced by intercurrent infection. Likewise, at least two viral loads, from the same laboratory using the same assay, should be obtained to avoid interassay variation.

The effect of prophylaxis against opportunistic infections, e.g. cotrimoxazole for *Pneumocystis jirovecii* pneumonia (PCP) and toxoplasmosis, has been shown to delay the onset of AIDS and change the pattern of disease manifestations. The CD4 count is the most important prognostic indicator in determining the likelihood of particular opportunistic infections (see Table 5.1).

## Further reading

Centers for Disease Control. 1993 Revised Classification System for HIV infection and Expanded Surveillance Case Definition for AIDS among Adolescents and Adults. *MMWR* 1992; 41(RR17).

Health Protection Agency. 30 years on. *Health Protection Report* 2011; 5(22); (www.hpa.org.uk/hpr/archives/2011/news2211.htm).

Health Protection Agency. HIV in the United Kingdom: 2010 Report. *Health Protection Report* 4:26 (www.hpa.org.uk).

Health Protection Agency. Numbers accessing care: national overview. (www.hpa.org.uk/web/HPAweb&HPAwebStandard/HPAweb_C/1203064766492).

# CHAPTER 6

# Routine Assessment and Follow-up of the Newly Diagnosed HIV-positive Individual

*L. Waters[1] and D. Asboe[2]*

[1]Mortimer Market Centre, London, UK
[2]Chelsea and Westminster Hospital, London, UK

## OVERVIEW

- Clinical sites in which HIV testing is performed should ensure that they have clear patient pathways for ongoing support and care of the newly diagnosed HIV-positive individual
- All newly diagnosed patients should be reviewed by an HIV clinician within 2 weeks, sooner if they have symptoms or other acute needs
- HIV-positive individuals should be reassured regarding the impact of cART on health and life expectancy; most individuals can be advised to plan for a normal life
- Regular clinical monitoring is required to identify co-morbidities commonly encountered in HIV infection, to ensure HIV treatment efficacy for those on treatment and to screen for combination antiretroviral therapy drug toxicities
- Annual vaccination for influenza is recommended
- HIV-positive individuals should be encouraged to disclose their HIV status to their primary care physician. As patients survive into older age, many of their clinical needs will be best managed in primary care

## Introduction

In the UK more than 70% of HIV testing occurs within sexual health services but, in line with recent national guidance, more tests are being performed in primary care and other medical settings. The success of routine, opt-out testing is illustrated by the high uptake in antenatal services, and it is anticipated that normalization of testing across a broad range of services will echo this success. Point-of-care testing (POCT) further improves access to testing, both in medical and community settings.

It is crucial, as the number of individuals being tested increases, and the range of testing sites broadens, that HIV testing is supported by robust links to ongoing support and care; approximately 1 in 14 newly diagnosed individuals in the UK did not return to the testing clinic and although some attended other services, most remained lost to follow-up.

*ABC of HIV and AIDS*, Sixth Edition. Edited by Michael W. Adler,
Simon G. Edwards, Robert F. Miller, Gulshan Sethi and Ian G. Williams.
© 2012 Blackwell Publishing Ltd. Published 2012 by Blackwell Publishing Ltd.

Some individuals will be diagnosed in more urgent circumstances than others. Late presentation of HIV is a significant problem in the UK, and in 2009 approximately half of all adults were diagnosed late (CD4 cell count <350 cells/µL within 3 months of diagnosis). Those diagnosed during an acute HIV-related illness may have to deal with the HIV diagnosis, treatment of opportunistic infection and the need to commence cART in quick succession; women diagnosed in pregnancy have additional issues. Here the support and skill of the multidisciplinary team is particularly important in ensuring the physical and psychological well being of the individual.

## First assessment

The first assessment of a newly diagnosed individual provides the opportunity to discuss HIV, perform a thorough medical, psychological and social review and to request the investigations that will provide the baseline for future monitoring and intervention. At this visit the foundations for high-quality care are laid; the clinician has the opportunity to ascertain the patient's knowledge and evaluate their need for further information and support. In the UK, national guidelines recommend that all newly diagnosed patients are reviewed by an HIV clinician within 2 weeks, sooner if they have symptoms or other acute needs.

### History

A detailed medical, social and psychological history should be performed at baseline (Box 6.1). A thorough review of symptoms may guide targeted physical examination and additional investigations.

Additional assessment tools may be useful as indicated by the history, for example screening questionnaires for depression/anxiety.

### Examination

A full examination of all body systems is recommended; particular attention should be paid to thorough palpation for lymphadenopathy, careful skin and mucous membrane examination. All patients with a CD4 count less than 50 cells/µL should have dilated fundoscopy to exclude retinal pathology, particularly cytomegalovirus (CMV) retinitis. This should ideally be performed by an experienced ophthalmologist.

The following baseline measurements should be documented:

- weight, height and body mass index (BMI)
- blood pressure
- waist circumference and/or waist–hip ratio.

## Investigations

All newly diagnosed HIV-positive individuals should undergo confirmatory laboratory diagnosis of HIV infection, including discrimination between HIV-1 and HIV-2. Avidity assays may be available, depending on local surveillance, to determine whether infection is recent (within 3–6 months) or chronic (more than 6 months). These have been validated for epidemiological purposes; communication of results to patients must be cautious, emphasizing the degree of uncertainty.

Routine baseline investigations, as recommended in the BHIVA Routine Investigation and Monitoring Guidelines (2011), are summarized in Table 6.1.

Mental health disorders are common in HIV-infected individuals and confirmed mental health diagnoses are, themselves, a risk factor for HIV acquisition. Many aspects of living with HIV can impact on mental health. All patients should undergo a mental health assessment by a clinician and a specialist health advisor, with a low threshold for referral to counselling, psychology or psychiatry services as indicated.

HIV is associated with neurocognitive impairment, although, in most cases, it is asymptomatic or mild. Controversy remains regarding prevalence, aetiology and prognosis; there is a lack of consensus regarding value of screening and the most appropriate screening tool.

## Interventions and discussion

### Contact tracing and partner notification

Thorough contact tracing and partner notification is essential; careful documentation of this, and eventual outcomes, must be performed. A patient may wish to delay disclosure to partners; some delay may be acceptable if there is no urgency (i.e. no ongoing risk behaviour). Attempts to encourage and support disclosure and testing of contacts should be made regularly; if refusal continues then additional action may be required.

Some newly diagnosed individuals will have a known HIV-positive partner; for others, partner testing will be required. Support around disclosure and testing of their partner should be available. Testing of children is a sensitive area and specialist input should be sought.

### Safe sex and transmission

There should be a clearly documented discussion of the following issues:

- safer sex
- importance of STI screening
- indications for post-exposure prophylaxis (PEP) and when/how to access
- transmission risks including impact of concurrent STI
- the issue of 'reckless transmission' and litigation.

### Prognosis and general health

Newly diagnosed individuals should be reassured regarding the impact of cART on health and life expectancy; most individuals can be advised to plan for a normal life expectancy. General health measures should be emphasized, such as exercise, nutrition and smoking cessation, particularly as HIV is associated with an increased risk of many co-morbidities.

Patients travelling abroad should be counselled about simple precautions such as infection prophylaxis and water safety where appropriate.

### Social and occupational considerations

Newly diagnosed individuals should be given advice, including onward referral to other agencies if required, regarding support groups, employment rights and access to benefits; in the UK, HIV is covered by the 2005 Disability Discrimination Act.

**Table 6.1** Recommended investigations at initial assessment of an individual newly diagnosed with HIV infection (BHIVA Guidelines 2011).

| Category | Tests |
|---|---|
| HIV markers | CD4 T cell count (absolute and percentage) and HIV-1 plasma viral load; repeat to confirm baseline within 1–3 months<br>HIV-1 drug-resistance test and HIV-1 subtype determination |
| Biochemistry | Creatinine and estimated GFR calculation – MDRD preferred (not weight-based)<br>Liver function tests (bilirubin, albumin, GGT and ALT and/or AST)<br>Bone profile (corrected calcium, phosphate and alkaline phosphatase) |
| Haematology | Full blood count |
| Urinalysis | Dipstick for blood, protein and glucose<br>Urine protein–creatinine ratio |
| Metabolic assessment | Lipid profile (total cholesterol, HDL-cholesterol, total cholesterol/HDL ratio and triglycerides; repeated fasting if abnormal)<br>Glucose |
| Serology | Syphilis<br>Hepatitis A (total or IgG)*<br>Hepatitis B surface antigen (HBsAg), anti-core total antibody (anti-HBc) and anti-surface antibody* (anti-HBs)<br>Hepatitis C antibody (followed by hepatitis C RNA testing if antibody positive and confirmation of antibody positive status if RNA negative)<br>Toxoplasma IgG antibody (CD4 T-cell count <200 cells/$\mu$L)<br>Measles IgG antibody<br>Varicella IgG antibody (unless patient has a reliable history of chickenpox or zoster)<br>Rubella IgG antibody in women of child-bearing age*<br>Schistosoma serology (if longer than 1 month spent in sub-Saharan Africa) |
| TB screening (see Chapter 9) | Interferon gamma release assay (IGRA) testing is recommended for screening for latent infection. The decision to perform screening is dependent on a risk assessment based on country of origin, blood CD4 cell count and length of time on antiretroviral therapy. In addition, all HIV-positive close contacts of people who have infectious TB should be followed up and offered chemo-preventative therapy according to NICE guidelines (http://www.nice.org.uk/nicemedia/live/13422/53638/53638.pdf) |
| Stool sample | Ova/cysts/parasites (if from, or spent >1 month in, tropics) |
| Imaging | Chest radiograph is not recommended routinely (unless indicated by symptoms/signs) except in the following:<br>Increased tuberculosis risk (e.g. highly endemic group/area, known contact history)<br>Previous chest disease<br>Injecting drug users |
| Additional | Sexual health screen<br>Cervical cytology in female patients<br>Cardiovascular risk estimate (e.g. JBS-2; HIV-specific calculators available)<br>Fracture risk assessment (over 50 s) |

*If negative refer to British HIV Association Guidelines for Immunization of HIV-Infected Adults 2008. *HIV Med* 2008;9:795–848.
ALT, alanine aminotransferase; AST, aspartate aminotransferase; GFR, glomerular filtration rate; GGT, gamma-glutamyl transferase; MDRD, modification of diet in renal disease.

Patients whose occupation may be affected by their HIV status should be provided with the relevant information and, with consent, referred to their occupational health service.

## Immunization

Respiratory illnesses are more common in HIV-positive individuals irrespective of CD4 count. Influenza vaccination should be provided annually. Immunization with the 23 valent pneumococcal vaccine is recommended in all HIV-infected adults. As outlined in Table 6.1, individuals who are non-immune to hepatitis B, measles, rubella or varicella should be offered vaccination; those non-immune to hepatitis A should be vaccinated as indicated (e.g. hepatitis B/C co-infection, men who have sex with men and drug users). Varicella vaccine responses are best at CD4 counts above 400 cells/$\mu$L but consider vaccination if over 200 cells/$\mu$L. Combined measles/mumps/rubella (MMR) vaccine should be offered to those non-immune to measles and/or women of child-bearing age who with no rubella immunity, ideally at CD4 >200 cells/$\mu$L. Hepatitis B vaccine can be commenced at any CD4; optimal antibody response may not be achieved at low CD4 and repeat vaccination may be required.

For psychological support, see Chapter 21.

## Follow-up

After the first consultation, follow-up should be arranged at an interval dependent on the individual's symptoms, needs and immune status.

Ongoing monitoring guidance for ART-naïve individuals is summarized in Table 6.2. Two to four visits annually, dependent on CD4 count, are recommended. Monitoring patients on ART is more complex and needs to take into account the potential long-term toxicities of cART, including renal, liver and bone disease. Regular HIV viral loads are essential to ensure continued effectiveness and adherence to prescribed cART.

In the UK, approximately 80% of patients are taking cART. In this group the risk of opportunistic infection is rare. Issues more commonly encountered include co-morbidities associated with ageing and drug–drug interactions with cART. All patients should be encouraged to register with a GP if they have not done so already, and to disclose their HIV status. Most co-morbidity

**Table 6.2** Recommended assessments in cART-naïve HIV-infected individuals (BHIVA).

| Category | Tests | Test frequency |
|---|---|---|
| History | Symptom enquiry (physical, psychological) | Every visit |
| | Sexual history | 6 monthly |
| | Medical problems (including STI) | Every visit |
| | Vaccination history | Every visit |
| Examination | Weight, blood pressure, body mass index | Annually |
| | Targeted physical examination | As guided by symptoms |
| Investigations | FBC | Annually |
| | Creatinine, eGFR, LFT, glucose, lipids | Annually |
| | Urinalysis (including protein–creatinine ratio) | Annually |
| | CD4 > 450 | 4–6 monthly |
| | CD4 < 450 | 3–4 monthly |
| | HIV-1 plasma viral load | 6 monthly |
| | Hepatitis B (tests will depend on previous status) | Annual serology for all susceptible patients |
| | Hepatitis C antibody if previously negative | Annually (MSM and IDU) |
| | Hepatitis C RNA testing if cleared previous infection (spontaneously or after treatment) and are at ongoing risk of reinfection | Annually |
| | STS serology | Every visit (MSM) or Annually (others) |
| | Sexual health screen | Annual Offer (more frequent if risks) |
| | Cervical cytology | Annually |
| Assessments | Cardiovascular disease risk (12 monthly) | Annually |
| | Fracture risk in patients over 50 (FRAX score) | Every 3 years |

management and prescribing of concomitant medication should be orchestrated by general practice. HIV clinicians need the support of GPs in maintaining accurate records, managing co-morbidities and, where appropriate, offering enhanced screening and intervention.

Non-AIDS malignancies and *M. tuberculosis* account for a disproportionate level of significant ill health in patients with sustained HIV virological control. Systemic symptoms such as fever, night sweats and weight loss should prompt investigation to exclude these diagnoses. HIV-positive individuals, particularly MSM, are at significantly increased risk of anal cancer. Diversity of opinion exists as to best screening strategy. Regular assessment of anal symptoms is advised.

For follow-up consultations and other considerations see Box 6.2.

**Box 6.2 The follow-up assessment: essential elements of the follow up medical, social and psychological history**

- Symptom review
  - Physical
  - Psychological
- Current medical history
  - Check to see if patient has had any new diagnoses made elsewhere since last HIV follow up assessment
- Mental health assessment
  - Current mental health status
  - Admission to hospital
  - Suicide attempts/deliberate self-harm
- Medication history
  - It is important to regularly review ART to ensure its acceptability and tolerability. Adherence should be documented.
  - Check for potential drug interactions with antiretroviral therapy
  - Newly prescribed medication elsewhere
  - Over-the-counter medications
  - Herbal remedies
  - Recreational drug use
- Vaccination history and travel plans
- Children
  - Aim to ensure that any exposed children are tested for HIV infection
- Sexual and reproductive history
  - This should be regularly assessed as partners and pregnancy plans may change over time
  - Recent sexual activity including new partner/s.
  - If new partner, assess if aware of HIV status and advise on how to avoid onward infection including use of condoms and post exposure prophylaxis.
  - Current conception plans and contraception issues
  - Check that cervical screening up to date
- GP contact and disclosure
  - All individuals who have previously declined disclosure should be strongly encouraged to reconsider decision to disclose to their GP

## Further reading

British HIV Association Guidelines for the Routine investigation and monitoring of adult HIV-1-infected individuals (2011). See www.bhiva.org.

# CHAPTER 7

# Tumours in HIV

*M. Bower*

Chelsea and Westminster Hospital, London, UK

## OVERVIEW

- Three cancers are AIDS-defining illnesses: Kaposi sarcoma (KS), high-grade B-cell non-Hodgkin's lymphoma (including primary cerebral lymphoma) and invasive cervical cancer. There has been a significant decline in the incidence of these since the introduction of combination antiretroviral therapy (cART)
- Most patients with cutaneous KS will respond to cART alone although this may take 6–12 months. Chemotherapy (usually liposomal anthracyclines) is advocated for advanced cutaneous and visceral KS
- The prevalence of non-AIDS-defining malignancies appears to be rising in cohorts on cART due to prolonged survival
- Cancers associated with viral infections such as anal cancer, Hodgkin's disease and hepatocellular cancers are significantly more common in the age gender-matched general population

## Introduction

People living with HIV are at increased risk of developing various cancers. Many of these malignancies are associated with known oncogenic viruses and in the case of at least two AIDS-defining cancers (Kaposi sarcoma (KS) and non-Hodgkin's lymphoma (NHL)) the risk rises as the CD4 cell count falls; the introduction of combination antiretroviral therapy (cART) has led to a decline in the incidence of these tumours in populations with access to cART. The overall risk of all non-AIDS-defining cancers is increased two to three times in people living with HIV. In contrast, there has been no fall in the incidence of these non-AIDS-defining malignancies, and their prevalence appears to be rising in cohorts on cART due to prolonged survival.

## AIDS-defining malignancies

Three cancers are AIDS-defining illnesses: KS, high-grade B-cell NHL (including primary cerebral lymphoma) and invasive cervical cancer. Other malignancies also occur more frequently in HIV-positive people.

*ABC of HIV and AIDS*, Sixth Edition. Edited by Michael W. Adler,
Simon G. Edwards, Robert F. Miller, Gulshan Sethi and Ian G. Williams.
© 2012 Blackwell Publishing Ltd. Published 2012 by Blackwell Publishing Ltd.

## AIDS-related systemic lymphoma
### Epidemiology and histology
Systemic high-grade B-cell non-Hodgkin's lymphomas occur 60–100 times more commonly in people with HIV than in the matched general population. There has been a decline in incidence since the era of cART, although this fall is more marked for primary cerebral NHL than for systemic NHL. Approximately one-third of the tumours are Burkitt or Burkitt-like lymphomas (Figure 7.1) and two-thirds are diffuse large cell lymphomas (Figure 7.2).

### Clinical presentation
Half the cases of systemic NHL present with nodal disease, 30% with gastrointestinal disease and the remainder with other extranodal disease. Finally, 1% present as effusions without nodal mass of disease, and this variant, called primary effusion lymphoma, is associated with KS herpesvirus (Figure 7.3).

### Clinical management and prognosis
The treatment of systemic AIDS-related NHL involves the administration of combination anthracycline-based chemotherapy with intrathecal chemotherapy for those at risk of meningeal relapse. This should be given with concomitant cART and opportunistic infection prophylaxis. This management approach will result in durable complete remission in 50–60% of patients who will in effect be cured of their NHL.

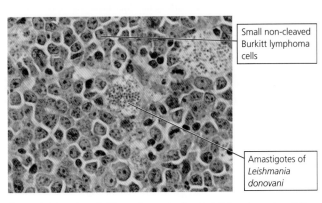

Small non-cleaved Burkitt lymphoma cells

Amastigotes of *Leishmania donovani*

**Figure 7.1** Lymph node biopsy demonstrating Burkitt lymphoma in addition to amastigotes of *Leishmania donovani*.

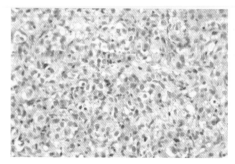

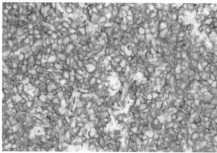

**Figure 7.2** Hepatic biopsy demonstrating diffuse large cell non-Hodgkin's lymphoma with immunostaining for CD20.

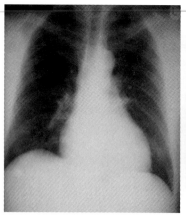

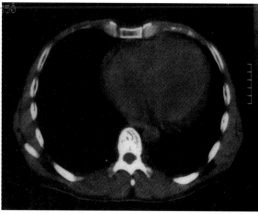

**Figure 7.3** Primary effusion lymphoma presenting with pericardial effusion.

## AIDS-related cerebral lymphoma

Primary cerebral lymphoma (PCL) is NHL that is confined to the craniospinal axis without systemic involvement. PCL is associated with advanced immunosuppression and has a particularly poor prognosis. The incidence of PCL has declined since the introduction of cART. Toxoplasmosis and PCL are the commonest causes of cerebral mass lesions in HIV and the differential diagnosis may prove difficult; both occur at low CD4 counts (<50 cells/$\mu$L) and present with headaches and focal neurological deficits. Clinical features that favour PCL include a more gradual onset over 2–8 weeks and the absence of a fever. Computed tomography (CT) and magnetic resonance imaging (MRI) scanning usually reveal solitary or multiple ring enhancing lesions with prominent mass effect and oedema. Again these features occur in both diagnoses, although PCL lesions are usually periventricular whereas toxoplasmosis more often affects the basal ganglia. More than 85% patients with cerebral toxoplasmosis will respond clinically and radiologically to 2 weeks of anti-toxoplasma therapy, and this has become the cornerstone of the diagnostic algorithm for cerebral mass lesions in severely immunodeficient patients. The detection of Epstein–Barr virus (EBV) DNA in the cerebrospinal fluid by polymerase chain reaction in patients with PCL has become established as a diagnostic test with a high sensitivity and specificity. [18]F-Flurodeoxyglucose positron emission tomography (FDG-PET) helps differentiate between PCL and cerebral toxoplasmosis (Figure 7.4).

## Clinical management and prognosis

The standard treatment modality for PCL in HIV patients is whole brain irradiation and in addition antiretroviral-naïve patients should start cART. Some clinicians advocate the use of intravenous chemotherapy for patients with PCL and a good performance status. Certainly a combination of systemic high-dose chemotherapy and radiotherapy has improved the survival of PCL in immunocompetent patients, and this approach has been used successfully in some HIV patients. However, the overall survival remains very poor (median survival 1–3 months).

## AIDS-related Kaposi sarcoma
### Epidemiology and histology

KS is caused by infection with a gammaherpesvirus named either Kaposi sarcoma herpesvirus (KSHV) or human herpesvirus 8 (HHV8). This virus is transmitted both horizontally and vertically. The highest levels of KSHV are found in saliva, and so kissing is thought to be a route of transmission.

Histologically KS is characterized by a proliferation of spindle-shaped cells accompanied by endothelial cells, fibroblasts and inflammatory cells that form slit-like vascular channels that resemble neo-angiogenesis (see Figure 7.5). The major clinical differential diagnosis is bacillary angiomatosis caused by the rickettsia *Bartonella henselae*, and this is best excluded by biopsy.

### Clinical presentation

Most patients with KS present with typical skin lesions that are typically multiple, pigmented, raised, painless and do not blanch (Figure 7.6). The earliest cutaneous lesions are frequently asymptomatic innocuous looking macular-pigmented lesions, which vary in colour from faint pink to vivid purple. Larger plaques occur usually on the trunk as oblong lesions following the line of skin

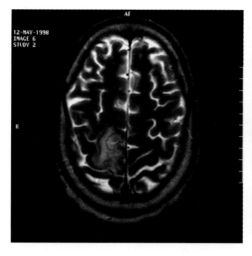
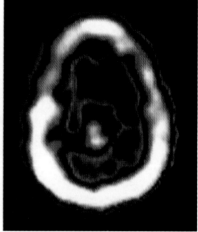

**Figure 7.4** Paired magnetic resonance imaging and $^{18}$F-flurodeoxyglucose positron emission tomography scans of a patient with AIDS-related primary cerebral lymphoma.

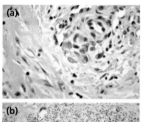

Early KS patch stage with small vessels with hyaline bodies within cells

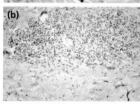

Plaque stage KS with presence of ill defined spindle cell proliferation forming small vascular spaces and associated with a mild chronic inflammatory cell infiltrate including plasma cells

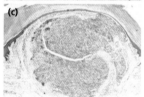

Nodular KS

**Figure 7.5** Histological stages of Kaposi sarcoma. (a) Early KS patch stage with small vessels with hyaline bodies within cells. (b) Plaque stage KS with presence of ill defined spindle cell proliferation forming small vascular spaces and associated with a mild chronic inflammatory cell infiltrate including plasma cells. (c) Nodular KS.

creases. Lesions may develop to form large plaques and nodules that can be associated with painful oedema. In addition to a thorough skin examination, inspection of the oral cavity and conjunctivae should be undertaken (Figure 7.7). Oral lesions are a frequent accompaniment that may lead to ulceration, dysphagia and secondary infection. A nodular form of KS that is frequently associated with lymphoedema is seen more commonly in people of African descent and often proves particularly difficult to control (Figure 7.8).

The most common sites of visceral KS are the lungs and stomach. Pulmonary KS is a life-threatening complication that usually presents with dyspnoea, dry cough, with or without fever and may cause haemoptysis. A chest radiograph typically reveals a diffuse reticulonodular infiltrate and pleural effusion (Figure 7.9). Gastrointestinal lesions are usually asymptomatic but may bleed or cause obstruction. The diagnosis is usually confirmed at endoscopy (Figure 7.10).

## Clinical management and prognosis

The clinical management of AIDS-associated KS is determined to a large extent by the clinical staging which is shown in Table 7.1.

**Table 7.1** The modified AIDS Clinical Trials Group staging of Kaposi sarcoma (1997).

| | Good risk (all of the following) T0I0 | Poor risk (any of the following) T1I1 |
|---|---|---|
| Tumour (T) | Confined to skin, lymph nodes or minimal oral disease | Tumour-associated oedema or ulceration<br>Extensive oral KS<br>Gastrointestinal KS<br>KS in other non-nodal viscera |
| Immune status (I) | CD4 count >150 cells/µL | CD4 <150 cells/µL |

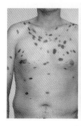
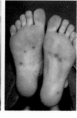
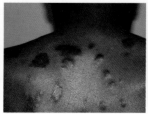
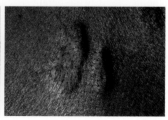

(a)

(b)

**Figure 7.6** (a, b) Cutaneous Kaposi sarcoma lesions.

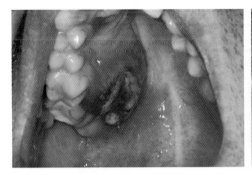

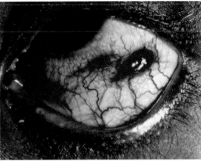

**Figure 7.7** Common non-cutaneous sites.

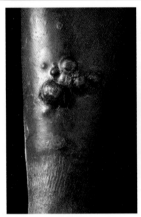

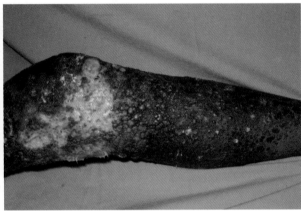

**Figure 7.8** Nodular Kaposi sarcoma.

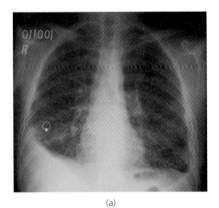

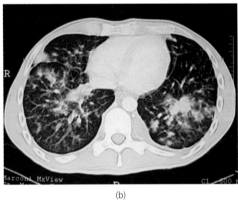

(a)                              (b)

**Figure 7.9** Pulmonary Kaposi sarcoma (chest radiograph (a) and computed tomography scan (b)).

Patients with T0 disease should commence cART. For most patients the KS will respond to cART alone, although this may take 6–12 months. In view of this delay, cosmetically significant localized lesions may be treated with either intralesional vinblastine or localized radiotherapy. Chemotherapy is advocated for advanced cutaneous and visceral KS (stage T1) but is not merited for early disease in view of the potential responses to cART. Liposomal anthracyclines are considered first-line chemotherapy for advanced KS, and paclitaxel chemotherapy is recommended for anthracycline-resistant disease. KS is no longer associated with an ominous prognosis, although patients with pulmonary involvement still only have a median survival of around 18 months.

## AIDS related cervical cancer
### Epidemiology and histology

Invasive cervical cancer has been included as an AIDS-defining diagnosis since 1993 and the precursor lesions, cervical intraepithelial neoplasia (CIN) or squamous intraepithelial lesion (SIL) occur more frequently in women with HIV. Human papilloma virus (HPV) has a central role in the pathogenesis, and HIV is associated with a high prevalence of HPV in the cervix, a high frequency of multiple HPV genotypes and persistence of HPV in the cervix, a high progression from low-grade SIL to high-grade SIL and likelihood of relapse of CIN II/III after therapy. The risk of SIL is greatest among women with CD4 cell counts <200 cells/μL and

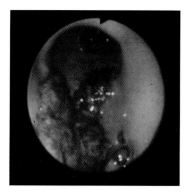

**Figure 7.10** Gastric Kaposi sarcoma (endoscopic appearances).

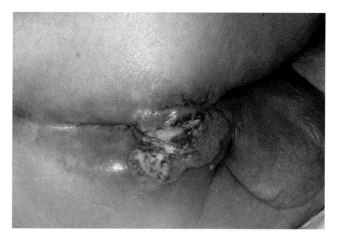

**Figure 7.11** Locally advanced anal cancer.

may regress with cART. These findings mandate close colposcopic surveillance.

### Clinical presentation and management

HIV-positive women with cervical cancer generally have more advanced stage disease at presentation. The management of invasive cervical cancer in HIV-positive women is the same as in the general population.

## Non-AIDS-defining malignancies

Overall, cancer occurs two to three times more commonly in HIV-positive people than the age- and gender-matched general population. Some tumours occur at much higher rates than others, including cancers associated with viral infections such as anal cancer, Hodgkin's disease and hepatocellular cancers. However, some cancers with no known viral aetiology such as seminoma and non-small cell lung cancers also occur significantly more commonly.

### HIV-related anal cancer
#### Epidemiology and histology

There is an increased incidence of anal carcinoma among HIV-positive patients but it is not an AIDS-defining diagnosis. The incidence of anal cancer among men who have sex with men (MSM) is estimated to be 35/100 000, which resembles the incidence of cervical cancer before the introduction of routine cervical screening. Anal cancer is twice as common in HIV-positive MSM as it is in HIV-negative MSM.

Anal cancer shares many features with cervical cancer, including association with HPV infection. High-grade squamous intraepithelial lesion (HSIL) or anal intraepithelial neoplasia (AIN) of the anus is believed to progress to invasive anal cancer in a fashion analogous to the progression from cervical HSIL or cervical CIN to invasive cervical cancer.

### Clinical presentation and management

Patients typically present with pain, bleeding and a mass (Figure 7.11). There is no clear correlation between risk of anal cancer and CD4 count. Combined modality therapy (CMT) of

chemotherapy with radiation treatment can result in tumour ablation with sphincter preservation. Most tumours can be controlled locally, with 5-year survival rates in the range of 65%, although the toxicity appears to be greater than in the HIV-negative population and salvage surgery may be necessary.

The future of anal cancer in HIV-seropositive people may lie with effective screening of the at-risk population and early intervention (Figure 7.12). Anal cytology and high-resolution anoscopy have been found to be effective methods of screening for AIN, and if therapeutic interventions could be shown to reduce progression and mortality this would be an attractive strategy. Some guidelines currently recommend regular digital examinations for HIV-positive MSM.

### HIV-related Hodgkin lymphoma
#### Epidemiology and histology

The incidence of Hodgkin's lymphoma (HD) is around 10 times higher in individuals with HIV, although HD is not an AIDS-defining diagnosis. EBV has been implicated in the pathogenesis, and the histological subtypes in patients with HIV are often less favourable.

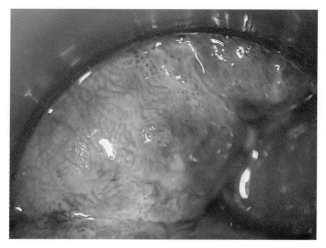

**Figure 7.12** Anoscopy appearance showing small ulcerated area of AIN 3.

Box 7.1 **Definition of an HIV associated MCD attack**

**1** Fever

**2** At least three of the following symptoms:

- Peripheral lymphadenopathy
- Enlarged spleen
- Oedema
- Pleural effusion
- Ascites
- Cough
- Nasal obstruction
- Xerostomia
- Rash
- Central neurologic symptoms
- Jaundice
- Autoimmune haemolytic anaemia

**3** Increased serum C-reactive protein level >20 mg/L in the absence of any other aetiology

*Source:* Gerard *et al.* (2007).

## Clinical presentation and management

Patients usually present with advanced stage disease and B symptoms, bone marrow infiltration and extranodal disease are all common. The optimal chemotherapy schedule for HIV-HD has not been determined. However, ABVD, Stanford V and hybrid regimens have been used. Since the era of cART the remission rates and overall survival have improved and approach those seen in the general population when matched for stage and other prognostic variables.

## HIV-related multicentric Castleman's disease
### Epidemiology and histology

Multicentric Castleman's disease (MCD) is a relatively rare lymphoproliferative disorder that is related to KSHV and the diagnosis is established histologically.

### Clinical presentation and management

Patients present with fever, lymphadenopathy and hepatosplenomegaly and a number of systemic symptoms (Box 7.1). High levels of HHV-8 DNA is almost always present in blood. Although there is no definitive gold standard treatment, the introduction of rituximab (an anti-CD20 antibody) in the era of cART has led to high overall survival rates.

## Further reading

BHIVA. AIDS Malignancy Guidelines. *HIV Med* 2008;9:681–720.

EACS. HIV Co-morbidity Guidelines. 2010 (www.europeanaidsclinicalsociety .org/guidelinespdf/2_Non_Infectious_Co_Morbidities_in_HIV.pdf).

Gerard L, Berezne A, Galicier L, *et al.* Prospective Study of rituximab in chemotherapy-dependent human immunodeficiency virus associated multicentric Castleman's disease: ANRS 117 Castlemab Trial. *J Clin Oncol* 2007; 25:3350–3356.

# CHAPTER 8

# The Lung and HIV

*S. Doffman[1] and R. F. Miller[2]*

[1]Brighton and Sussex University Hospitals, Brighton, UK
[2]University College London, London, UK

## OVERVIEW

- 60% of HIV-infected individuals will experience at least one significant episode of respiratory disease during their lifetime
- Bacterial pneumonia occurs six to 10 times more frequently in HIV-infected subjects not taking cART than with the HIV-uninfected general population
- *Pneumocystis* pneumonia (PCP) is one of the most common opportunistic infections and has a mortality rate of approximately 10%. PCP prophylaxis should be given to all patients with a CD4 count <200 cells/μL
- Palatal Kaposi sarcoma strongly predicts the presence of pulmonary and/or foregut disease
- Bronchoscopy is an important investigation when diagnosing HIV-associated respiratory tract conditions

The lungs are commonly affected in HIV-positive individuals. A wide variety of illnesses and pathogens can be encountered. This chapter will focus on common causes of HIV-related lung disease (Box 8.1). In HIV-infected subjects with reasonably preserved immunity (normal or near normal CD4 counts), typical community-acquired infections occur but at greater frequency than in the general population. With advancing HIV-induced immunosuppression (CD4 counts <200 cells/μL), the risk of opportunistic infections and malignancy increases.

While HIV treatment leads to significant reductions in the incidence of HIV-associated opportunistic infections and malignancies, respiratory problems remain a major cause of disease.

## Infections

### Bacterial infection

Upper respiratory tract infections, acute bronchitis and acute and symptomatic chronic sinusitis occur more frequently in HIV-infected patients than in the general population.

### Bronchitis

The presentation mimics exacerbations of chronic obstructive lung disease; most patients have a productive cough and fever. Commonly identified pathogens are *Streptococcus pneumoniae* and *Haemophilus influenzae*.

### Box 8.1 **HIV-associated respiratory disease**

**Infections**

- Acute bronchitis
- Acute sinusitis
- Chronic sinusitis
- Bronchiectasis
- Bacterial pneumonia
- Tuberculosis
- *Pneumocystis jirovecii* pneumonia
- *Cryptococcus neoformans* pneumonia
- *Histoplasma capsulatum*
- Influenza A

**Malignancy**

- Cytomegalovirus
- Kaposi sarcoma

**Non-malignant conditions**

- Lung cancer
- Non-specific interstitial pneumonitis
- Lymphoctic interstitial pneumonitis
- Chronic obstructive pulmonary disease
- Pulmonary arterial hypertension
- Pneumothorax

### Bronchiectasis

Bronchiectasis is increasingly recognized among patients with advanced HIV disease and low CD4 lymphocyte counts. It probably arises secondary to recurrent bacterial, mycobacterial or *Pneumocystis jirovecii* infection. The diagnosis is made by high-resolution computed tomography scanning (Figure 8.1).

### Pneumonia

Bacterial pneumonia occurs six to 10 times more frequently in HIV-infected subjects not taking cART than in the HIV-uninfected general population. It is especially common in HIV-infected

*ABC of HIV and AIDS*, Sixth Edition. Edited by Michael W. Adler,
Simon G. Edwards, Robert F. Miller, Gulshan Sethi and Ian G. Williams.
© 2012 Blackwell Publishing Ltd. Published 2012 by Blackwell Publishing Ltd.

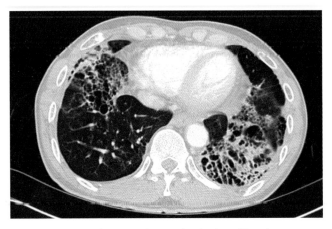

**Figure 8.1** Computed tomography scan showing bronchiectasis.

injecting drug users. The widespread use of cART has led to a reduction in rates of bacterial pneumonia and bacteraemia but they are still considerably higher than those seen in the non-HIV-infected general population. The spectrum of bacterial pathogens is similar to that in non-HIV-infected individuals. *S. pneumoniae* is the commonest cause, followed by *H. influenzae*. Infection with *Staphylococcus aureus* and Gram-negative organisms may occur in advanced HIV disease. *Mycoplasma*, *Legionella* and *Chlamydia* species do not appear to be more frequent. HIV-infected individuals with *S. pneumoniae* pneumonia are frequently bacteraemic.

Bacterial pneumonia has a similar clinical presentation in HIV-infected and uninfected individuals. Chest radiographs are frequently atypical, mimicking *Pneumocystis* pneumonia (PCP) in

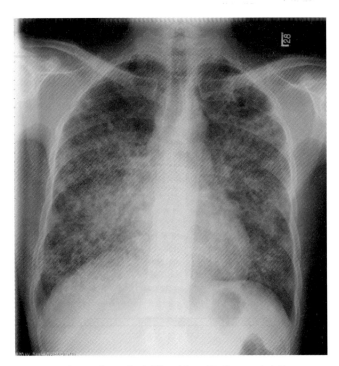

**Figure 8.2** Chest radiograph of diffuse bilateral infiltrates mimicking *Pneumocystis jirovecii* pneumonia, due to *Streptococcus pneumoniae*.

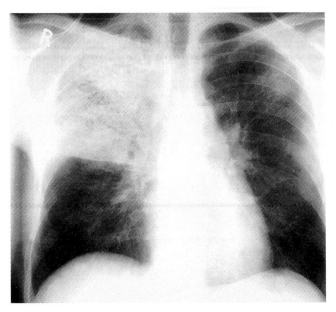

**Figure 8.3** Chest radiograph of lobar pneumonia due to *Streptococcus pneumoniae*.

up to half of cases (Figure 8.2). Lobar or segmental consolidation may occur with a wide range of bacterial organisms, including *S. pneumoniae*, *P. aeruginosa*, *H. influenzae* and *Mycobacterium tuberculosis* (Figure 8.3).

Treatment of bacterial pneumonia in HIV-infected patients should be as in HIV-uninfected individuals, using British or American Thoracic Society guidelines. The same clinical and laboratory prognostic indices described for the general population apply to HIV-infected patients. Expert microbiological advice on local antibiotic resistance patterns should be sought as treatment is usually begun on an empirical basis. Complications include intrapulmonary cavitation, abscess formation and empyema. There is a high relapse rate, despite appropriate antibiotic therapy.

Immunization with 23-valent pneumococcal vaccine is recommended in all adults and adolescents (at diagnosis of HIV infection and after 5 years), although humoral responses and clinical efficacy are probably impaired in those with CD4 counts <200 cells/μL.

## Fungal infection
### Pneumocystis pneumonia

*Pneumocystis jirovecii*, formerly called *Pneumocystis carinii*, is the cause of *Pneumocystis* pneumonia (the acronym PCP still applies, *Pneumocystis* pneumonia). It remains a common presentation in individuals unaware of their HIV serostatus and also among HIV-infected patients intolerant of, or non-adherent with, PCP prophylaxis and/or cART.

Patients present with non-productive cough and progressive exertional breathlessness of several days to weeks duration, with or without fever. On auscultation the chest is usually clear; occasionally, end-inspiratory crackles are audible. In early PCP the chest radiograph may be normal (~10% cases). The most common abnormality is bilateral, perihilar interstitial infiltrates (Figure 8.4),

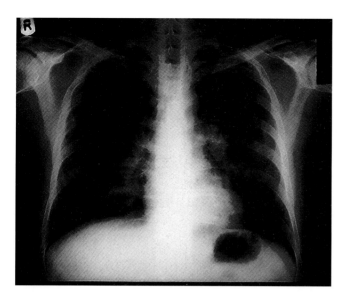

**Figure 8.4** Chest radiograph of *Pneumocystis jirovecii* pneumonia – diffuse bilateral infiltrates.

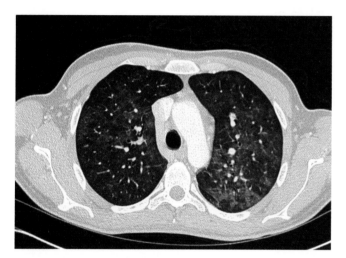

**Figure 8.5** Computed tomography scan of the thorax showing diffuse bilateral patchy 'ground glass' shadowing in *Pneumocystis jirovecii* pneumonia.

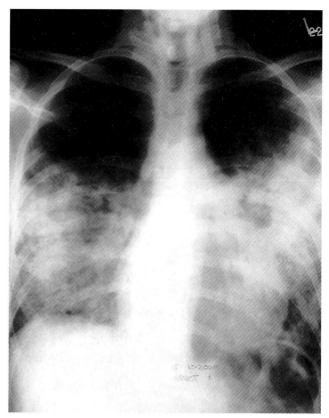

**Figure 8.6** Chest radiograph of showing marked diffuse bilateral abnormalities due to severe *Pneumocystis* pneumonia.

This stratification is useful as oral therapy may be given to those with mild disease. First-choice treatment for PCP of all severity is high-dose co-trimoxazole (sulfamethoxazole 100 mg/kg/day with trimethoprim 20 mg/kg/day) in two to four divided doses orally or intravenously for 21 days. Approximately 80% of patients will successfully complete this regimen. Treatment-limiting drug toxicity is common and <10% will not respond to treatment (defined by deterioration after $\geq$5 days of therapy).

which are more clearly seen on CT scanning (Figure 8.5) and which may progress to diffuse alveolar shadowing over a period of a few days (Figure 8.6). Atypical radiographic appearances include upper zone infiltrates resembling tuberculosis, hilar/mediastinal lymphadenopathy, intrapulmonary nodules and lobar consolidation, which are present in up to 20%.

Treatment is usually started empirically in patients with typical clinical and radiological features and a CD4 count of <200 cells/$\mu$L, or clinical stigmata of immune deficiency, e.g. oral hairy leucoplakia or cutaneous Kaposi sarcoma (KS), pending diagnosis by cytological analysis of bronchoalveolar lavage (BAL) fluid or induced sputum samples (Figure 8.7).

Several factors predict poor outcome from PCP (Box 8.2).

PCP can be stratified clinically as *mild* ($PaO_2 > 11.0$ kPa), *moderate* ($PaO_2 = 8.0$–$11.0$ kPa) or *severe* ($PaO_2 < 8.0$ kPa) (Table 8.1).

---

**Box 8.2 Factors associated with a poor outcome from PCP**

**Factors present at, or soon after presentation**

- increasing patient age
- a second or third episode of PCP
- hypoxaemia (low $PaO_2$ or widened $A$-$aO_2$ gradient)
- low haemoglobin
- low albumin
- raised serum bilirubin
- raised CRP
- coexistent pulmonary Kaposi sarcoma
- coexistent medical co-morbidity, e.g. lymphoma or pregnancy

**Once hospitalized**

- development of pneumothorax
- admission to the intensive care unit
- need for mechanical ventilation

**Table 8.1** Stratification of severity of *Pneumocystis jirovecii* pneumonia.

| | Mild | Moderate | Severe |
|---|---|---|---|
| Symptoms and signs | Dyspnoea on exertion, with or without cough and sweats | Dyspnoea on minimal exertion and occasionally at rest; cough and fever | Dyspnoea and tachypnoea at rest; persistent fever and cough |
| Oxygenation | | | |
| PaO$_2$, breathing room air, at rest (kPa) | >11.0 | 8.1–11.0 | ≤8.0 |
| SaO$_2$, breathing room air, at rest (%) | >96 | 91–96 | <91 |
| SaO$_2$, breathing room air, on exercise (%) | >90 | <90 | <90 |
| A-aO$_2$ (kPa) | <4.7 | 4.7–6.0 | >6.0 |
| Chest radiograph | Normal or minor perihilar shadowing | Diffuse bilateral interstitial shadowing | Extensive interstitial shadowing with or without diffuse alveolar shadowing |

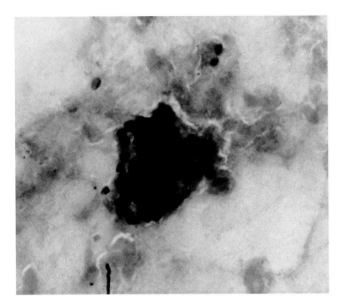

**Figure 8.7** Demonstration of *Pneumocystis jirovecii* in bronchoalveolar lavage fluid; Grocott methenamine silver stain.

In patients who develop toxicity or do not respond to co-trimoxazole, alternative therapy in severe disease is clindamycin (450–600 mg qds orally or intravenous) plus oral primaquine (15 mg daily) or intravenous pentamidine (4 mg/kg daily) (see Table 8.2 for alternatives).

Patients with an admission PaO$_2$ ≤9.3 kPa (<70 mmHg) or an A-aO$_2$ of >4.7 kPa (>33 mmHg) should also receive adjuvant glucocorticoids within 72 hours of starting specific anti-PCP treatment (see Chapter 20). This has been shown to reduce the need for mechanical ventilation and reduce mortality.

## Intensive care

Over the last decade the prognosis for patients with severe PCP and respiratory failure requiring admission to the intensive care unit (ICU) has improved. This is probably because of better ICU management of respiratory failure and acute lung injury, rather than to specific improvements in PCP care or to cART. Factors associated with poor outcome from PCP on the ICU include increasing patient age, need for mechanical ventilation and development of a pneumothorax.

Patients are at increased risk of PCP as their CD4 count decreases. Indications for prophylaxis are given in (Table 8.3).

Recommended regimens for PCP prophylaxis are listed in Table 8.4.

**Table 8.3** Indications for prophylaxis of PCP.

Primary prophylaxis
  CD4 count <200 cells/µl
  CD4 count <14% of total lymphocyte count
  History of another AIDS-defining diagnosis, e.g. Kaposi sarcoma

Secondary prophylaxis
  All patients after an episode of PCP

Discontinue secondary prophylaxis for patients on cART with
  Sustained increase in CD4 count >200 cells/µL AND
  Undetectable plasma HIV RNA
  (Both for ≥3 months)

**Table 8.2** Treatment of *Pneumocystis jirovecii* pneumonia.

| Disease severity | Mild | Moderate | Severe |
|---|---|---|---|
| First choice | Co-trimoxazole | Co-trimoxazole | Co-trimoxazole |
| Alternative therapy | Clindamycin–primaquine or Dapsone with trimethoprim or Atovaquone | Clindamycin–primaquine or Dapsone with trimethoprim or Atovaquone | Clindamycin–primaquine or Intravenous pentamidine |

**Table 8.4** Regimens for prophylaxis of PCP.

| | Drug | Dose | Note |
|---|---|---|---|
| First choice | Co-trimoxazole | 960 mg or 480 mg od or 960 mg × 3/week | |
| Second choice | Nebulized pentamidine | 300 mg × 1/month via jet nebulizer | Use × 1/fortnight if CD4 count <50 cells/µL |
| | Dapsone and pyrimethamine | 100 mg od 25 mg × 3/week | |
| Third choice | Atovaquone | 750 mg bd | |

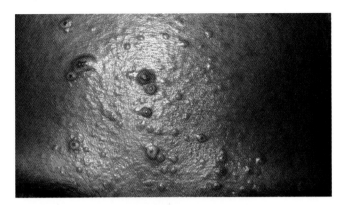

**Figure 8.8** Cutaneous lesions in disseminated cryptococcosis.

## Cryptococcal infection

Pulmonary infection presents either as primary cryptococcosis (which has a non-specific presentation), or as part of a disseminated infection with meningitis with/without cryptococcaemia (Figure 8.8). Examination of the chest is normal or reveals crackles. Radiographic abnormalities include focal or diffuse interstitial infiltrates; focal masses, mediastinal or hilar lymphadenopathy, nodules or effusion. Diagnosis of pulmonary infection is by identification of *Cryptococcus neoformans* in respiratory secretions or lung tissue (Figure 8.9). Treatment is with fluconazole, or with liposomal amphotericin and flucytosine.

## Histoplasmosis

Pulmonary histoplasmosis invariably occurs as part of a disseminated infection. Patients typically have a subacute presentation with fever and weight loss; approximately half have a non-productive cough and dyspnoea. Examination frequently shows hepatosplenomegaly. The chest radiograph is normal or shows bilateral, widespread ≤4 mm nodules in approximately a third of cases. Alveolar consolidation, interstitial infiltrates and reticulonodular shadowing have been described. The diagnosis is made identifying the organism in BAL fluid, or lung tissue. Serum $(1–3)$-β-D-glucan levels may be elevated but are non-specific. Liposomal amphotericin is the preferred treatment for those severely unwell. Itraconazole is an option for milder disease.

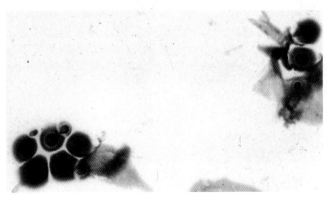

**Figure 8.9** *Cryptococcus neoformans* in bronchoalveolar lavage fluid.

## Aspergillus infection

Pulmonary infection with *Aspergillus* is uncommon in HIV-positive individuals. Risk factors are neutropenia and corticosteroid therapy. Presentation is non-specific; fever, cough and dyspnoea are common, but pleuritic chest pain and haemoptysis also occur. Radiographic abnormalities are non-specific. Diagnosis is by identification of *Aspergillus* in respiratory secretions or lung tissue. Serum $(1–3)$-β-D-glucan levels may be elevated (but are non-specific). Treatment is with voriconazole, or liposomal amphotericin.

## Viral infection
### Influenza A

Influenza A does not occur more commonly in HIV-infected individuals but appears to have a greater risk of more severe disease (Figure 8.10). In both seasonal and H1N1 influenza the typical presentation is with coryzal symptoms, fever, headache and myalgia. In some HIV-infected patients especially those with CD4 cell counts <100 cells/μL the illness may deteriorate rapidly and may be complicated by secondary bacterial pneumonia. The diagnosis is made by detection of viral antigen or RNA in a nasopharyngeal aspirate or nasal swab. As in the general population, HIV-infected patients presenting with documented or suspected influenza A and duration of symptoms ≤48 hours should receive a neuraminidase inhibitor, e.g. oseltamivir.

### Cytomegalovirus

CMV is frequently isolated in BAL fluid from symptomatic patients with CD4 counts <100 cells/μL, and who have another diagnosis, e.g. PCP. However in this context it is unclear whether CMV is causing disease. In patients where CMV is the sole identified pathogen, clinical presentation and chest radiographic abnormalities are non-specific. CMV pneumonitis is diagnosed by identifying characteristic intranuclear and intracytoplasmic inclusions in BAL fluid cells or in lung tissue.

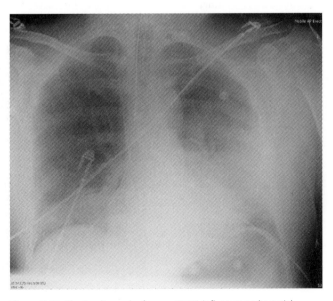

**Figure 8.10** Chest radiograph of severe H1N1 influenza; no bacterial copathogen.

## Tuberculosis
See Chapter 9.

## Malignant conditions

### Kaposi sarcoma
Pulmonary KS is almost always accompanied by cutaneous or lymphadenopathic KS. Palatal KS strongly predicts the presence of pulmonary and/or foregut disease. Presentation is with non-specific cough and progressive dyspnoea; haemoptysis is less common.

Within the thorax, KS may involve the airways, lung parenchyma, pleura and mediastinal lymph nodes. Radiological findings include interstitial or nodular infiltrates and alveolar consolidation; pleural effusion is seen in up to 40% and hilar/mediastinal lymphadenopathy occurs in ~25% of patients (Figure 8.11).

Diagnosis is confirmed at bronchoscopy in >50% cases by the appearance of multiple, raised or flat, red or purple endotracheal and endobronchial lesions. Biopsy is rarely done since cutaneous KS is usually present and the diagnostic yield from biopsy is <20%. cART may induce remission of pulmonary KS and is used in addition to chemotherapy.

### Bronchial carcinoma
Lung cancer appears to be two to four times more common in HIV-infected smokers. It is now more frequently diagnosed than in the pre-cART era. Presentation is usually with disseminated disease, and the prognosis is therefore poor (Figure 8.12).

## Non-malignant, non-infectious conditions

### Non-specific pneumonitis
Non-specific pneumonitis mimics PCP but often occurs at higher blood CD4 counts. Diagnosis is made by transbronchial, VATS (video-assisted thoracoscopic surgery) or open-lung biopsy. Most episodes are self-limiting, but prednisolone may be beneficial.

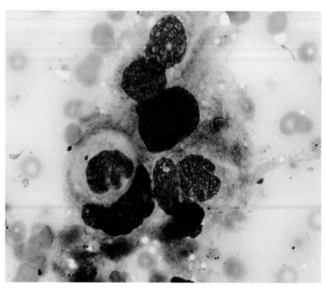

**Figure 8.12** Cytological smear showing squamous cell carcinoma. Sample obtained via EBUS-guided biopsy of a mediastinal lymph node.

### Lymphocytic interstitial pneumonitis
Lymphocytic interstitial pneumonitis is more commonly seen in HIV-infected children and clinically resembles idiopathic pulmonary fibrosis. Presentation is with slowly progressive dyspnoea and cough, symptoms that are indistinguishable from infection. Chest examination may be normal or reveal fine end-inspiratory crackles. The chest radiograph usually shows bilateral reticulonodular infiltrates but may show diffuse shadowing mimicking PCP. Diagnosis requires biopsy. Treatment with cART is often effective.

### Chronic obstructive pulmonary disease
HIV-infected smokers are at increased risk of developing chronic obstructive lung disease (Figure 8.13). The synergistic effects of

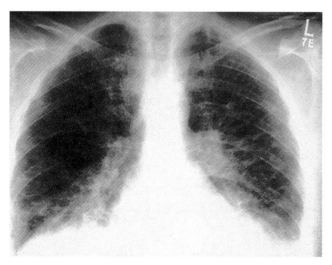

**Figure 8.11** Chest radiograph of Kaposi sarcoma, pleural effusions.

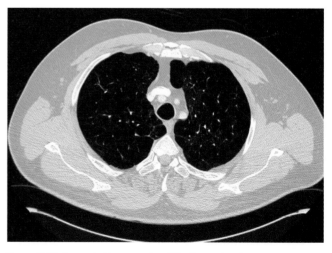

**Figure 8.13** Computed tomography of the thorax showing severe emphysema.

cigarette smoking, recurrent bacterial and opportunistic infections, injecting drug use and possibly direct effects of HIV in the lung argue strongly for promoting smoking cessation services for HIV-infected patients.

## Pulmonary arterial hypertension

Pulmonary arterial hypertension is reported to be six to 12 times more common in HIV-infected populations. The presentation and management are similar to that among non-HIV-infected individuals. cART is associated with improved haemodynamics and survival.

## Pneumothorax

Pneumothorax occurs more frequently in HIV-infected patients when compared with the age-matched general medical population. Risk factors include cigarette smoking and receipt of nebulized pentamidine. PCP should be excluded in any patient presenting with a pneumothorax.

## Further reading

Crothers K, Thompson BW, Burkhardt K, *et al.* Lung HIV Study. HIV-associated lung infections and complications in the era of combination antiretroviral therapy. *Proc Am Thorac Soc* 2011;8:275–281.

Huang L, Cattamanchi A, Davis JL, *et al.* International HIV-Associated Opportunistic Pneumonias (IHOP) Study; Lung HIV Study. HIV-associated Pneumocystis pneumonia. *Proc Am Thorac Soc* 2011;8:294–300.

Kaplan JE, Benson C, Holmes KH, *et al.* Centers for Disease Control and Prevention (CDC); National Institutes of Health; HIV Medicine Association of the Infectious Diseases Society of America. Guidelines for prevention and treatment of opportunistic infections in HIV-infected adults and adolescents: recommendations from CDC, the National Institutes of Health, and the HIV Medicine Association of the Infectious Diseases Society of America. *MMWR Recomm Rep* 2009;58(RR-4):1–207.

Morris A, Crothers K, Beck JM, Huang L. American Thoracic Society Committee on HIV Pulmonary Disease. An official ATS workshop report: Emerging issues and current controversies in HIV-associated pulmonary diseases. *Proc Am Thorac Soc* 2011;8:17–26.

Pozniak A, Coyne K, Miller R, *et al.* on behalf of the BHIVA Guidelines Subcommittee. British HIV Association guidelines for the treatment of TB/HIV coinfection 2011. *HIV Medicine* 2011;12:517–524.

# CHAPTER 9

# HIV and Tuberculosis Co-infection

*F. Perrin[1], R. Breen[2] and M. Lipman[3]*

[1]King's College Hospital, London, UK
[2]Guy's and St Thomas' Hospital, London, UK
[3]Royal Free Hospital, University College London, London, UK

## OVERVIEW

- HIV is a key driver of the global rise in tuberculosis (TB) cases through accelerated progression of TB and greatly increased risk of reactivation
- TB/HIV has a wide range of clinical presentations, many with non-specific symptoms and signs – leading to potential diagnostic delay
- Standard regimens of anti-TB drugs can be successfully combined with combination antiretroviral therapy (cART) to achieve good outcomes for both TB (similar to HIV-uninfected individuals) and HIV (similar to those without TB)
- cART should generally be started early (i.e. within the first few weeks or months) of anti-TB treatment in cART-naïve individuals
- Adverse events including immune reconstitution inflammatory syndrome are common but can be managed usually without interruption of either anti-HIV or anti-TB therapy
- Control of TB/HIV requires integration of TB detection and treatment with cART delivery programmes that minimize the development of drug resistance, adverse drug interactions and improve overall outcome

Tuberculosis (TB) and HIV infection are inextricably linked. Over the last 30 years, they have been responsible for an increasing global burden of death and disease. Despite the enormous challenge this presents to healthcare workers and policy-makers, there are now genuine grounds for optimism. Effective drug therapy can cure TB and combination antiretroviral therapy (cART) has reduced the risk of AIDS and death. Consequently, where such treatments are available the outlook for individuals diagnosed with HIV/TB co-infection is excellent.

## Background and epidemiology

The changes in innate and cellular immunity associated with HIV reduce the host's ability to control *Mycobacterium tuberculosis* (*M.tb*). This makes recent infection much more likely to rapidly progress to active disease and clinically latent *M.tb* infection (LTBI)

*ABC of HIV and AIDS*, Sixth Edition. Edited by Michael W. Adler, Simon G. Edwards, Robert F. Miller, Gulshan Sethi and Ian G. Williams.
© 2012 Blackwell Publishing Ltd. Published 2012 by Blackwell Publishing Ltd.

to reactivate. Whereas an HIV-uninfected individual with LTBI has a *lifetime* chance of reactivation of approximately 10%, those with HIV have an estimated risk closer to 10% *per annum*. Overall an HIV co-infected person is 20–40 times more likely to develop active TB. It is not surprising, therefore, that unlike other areas where TB incidence is falling, countries with a high HIV and TB overlap report increasing rates of TB. As discussed later, effective TB control can only be achieved if there is widespread implementation of cART. An estimated 12% (1.1 million) new TB cases each year worldwide are attributable to HIV – with this proportion being closer to one-third in sub-Saharan Africa (Figure 9.1). TB is the cause of around one-quarter of all adult AIDS deaths. The importance of offering an HIV test, and hence the opportunity for life-saving cART, to all patients diagnosed with TB, therefore, cannot be overemphasized.

## Presentation and diagnosis of active disease

A key component of TB control is the prompt recognition and diagnosis of active disease. A wide range of clinical features are associated with active TB/HIV, which in part results from the altered immune response present in advancing HIV infection. For example, as the blood CD4 count falls, the 'typical' chest radiographic feature of upper zone, cavitary disease is replaced by pulmonary infiltrates, mediastinal lymphadenopathy and pleural effusions (Figure 9.2a,b). Non-pulmonary, disseminated and multi-organ involvement is also more common (Figure 9.3).

Symptoms of TB such as fever, night sweats and weight loss are, if anything, more frequently seen in HIV co-infected patients. However, they can be misdiagnosed as arising from other causes including HIV itself. Conversely, it is increasingly reported from TB endemic areas that 5–20% of cases of (usually acid-fast bacilli (AFB) smear negative) culture-confirmed active pulmonary TB may have a normal or near-normal chest radiograph, and minimal systemic symptoms to suggest active disease. This makes screening for active TB using 'patient reported symptom scores' potentially less useful. It is unclear whether this form of subclinical active TB occurs to any great extent in areas of lower TB prevalence.

HIV co-infection does not alter the importance of the standard diagnostic methods of AFB smear and culture. However, HIV-positive subjects with pulmonary TB are more likely to be AFB sputum smear-negative – making this inexpensive and rapid test less

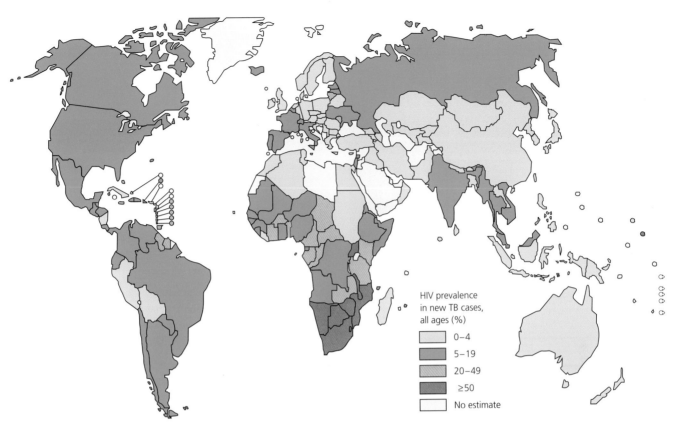

**Figure 9.1** Estimated HIV prevalence in new TB cases 2009 (WHO).

HIV prevalence
in new TB cases,
all ages (%)

| | 0–4 |
| | 5–19 |
| | 20–49 |
| | ≥50 |
| | No estimate |

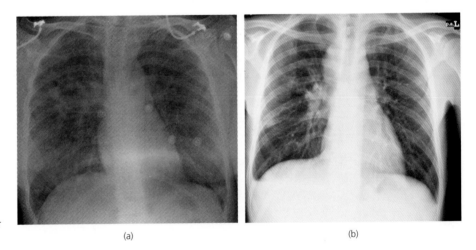

**Figure 9.2** Presentation of early TB/HIV. (a) Note in particular the right upper lobe thick-walled cavitation. (b) Note in particular the right paratracheal lymphadenopathy, lower zone infiltrate and right pleural effusion.

(a)　　　　(b)

sensitive. Given the high rate of disseminated and non-pulmonary disease, culture of samples other than sputum (such as blood and urine) can be helpful.

Novel and rapid tests to detect active TB regardless of disease site would be especially useful for HIV-infected individuals. The microscopic observation drug susceptibility assay (MODS), in which sputum is inoculated in anti-TB drug-free and drug-containing liquid media and examined microscopically for early growth, is a cheap, simple and rapid test (result in days) that appears to be sensitive and specific, and largely unaffected by HIV status. It also provides information on drug resistance; and has been shown to be of clinical value in a number of studies in resource-constrained environments worldwide. The recent introduction of nucleic acid amplification tests, which are both simple to use and provide a rapid result (in hours), that can also indicate significant resistance to key drugs such as rifampicin, isoniazid and fluoroquinolones is another important, although initially expensive, advance in TB diagnostics (Table 9.1).

The prevalence of drug-resistant TB is two- to threefold higher in HIV co-infected patients (Table 9.2). This is not thought to

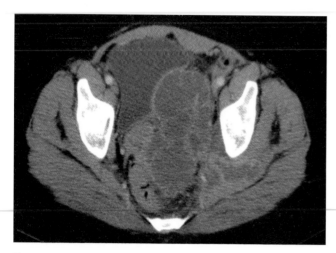

**Figure 9.3** Extrapulmonary tuberculosis. There is a huge, necrotic pelvic lymph node mass displacing the bladder and uterus.

**Table 9.1** The impact of HIV on clinical presentation and tests used to diagnose active disease or latent TB infection (LTBI).

| Feature or test | Effect of HIV |
| --- | --- |
| Clinical presentation | Often atypical |
| Chest radiograph | Often atypical: lacks characteristic upper zone distribution and cavitation; increased pulmonary infiltrates, mediastinal lymph nodes and pleural effusions |
| Sputum smear for AFB | More likely to be paucibacillary or negative |
| Sputum liquid culture | More likely to be negative |
| Nucleic acid amplification tests, e.g.<br>• XpertTB MTB/RIF<br>• GenoType MTBDRsl assay | Reduced sensitivity ~10–30% |
| MODS | Sensitivity (~80%) and specificity generally unaffected |
| Urine LAM | Low sensitivity in non-HIV infected (10–90%), increased in HIV positive (up to 50% improvement, especially with advanced disease) |
| Histology of tissue sample | Poorly formed granulomas with less caseation; less AFB present |
| TST | False negative in 20–40% cases of LTBI |
| Rapid immune-based tests, e.g.<br>• T spot TB<br>• Quantiferon Gold | Reduced sensitivity ~20% |

AFB, acid fast bacilli; LAM, lipoarabinomannan; MODS, microscopic observation drug susceptibility assay; TST, tuberculin skin test.

arise from an increased susceptibility to these strains; but more that HIV-infected subjects rapidly develop active disease, which, if involving a drug-resistant strain, can then be widely transmitted to others who may also be HIV infected. The latter will then themselves develop disease rapidly, and so the drug-resistant strain will appear more prevalent within the HIV population than others. This has an important clinical implication as, if drug resistance is not

**Table 9.2** Definitions of *Mycobacterium tuberculosis* drug resistance.

| | Definition | Effect of HIV |
| --- | --- | --- |
| Monoresistant TB | Resistance to one drug | Most commonly isoniazid resistance; HIV associated with increased incidence of rifampicin resistance |
| Multiple drug resistant (MDR) TB | Resistance to isoniazid and rifampicin | Worse outcome through rapid progression of disease |
| Extensively drug resistant (XDR) TB | MDR + fluoroquinolone resistance + resistance to at least one of three second line injectable agents (capreomycin, kanamycin, amikacin) | Worse outcome through rapid progression of disease |

suspected promptly, potentially fatal undertreatment may occur. An extreme example of this was the first large-scale description of extensively drug-resistant (XDR) TB linked to HIV co-infection in South Africa, where mortality was around 50% within 1 month of diagnostic suspicion of disease.

## Treatment

HIV co-infection does not alter the standard and reliable anti-TB regimens which can achieve generally high rates of cure and low relapse similar to those found in HIV-uninfected subjects. Pulmonary or extrapulmonary TB without cerebral involvement, in the first instance pending drug sensitivity information, should receive rifampicin, isoniazid, pyrazinamide and ethambutol for 2 months followed by rifampicin and isoniazid for a further 4 months. Some experts suggest extending this for severe disease such as extensive pulmonary cavitation or widespread dissemination. To ensure adequate drug delivery and adherence, regimens are often delivered in fixed-dose combinations, daily or three-times weekly according to local practice (which may be self-administered or directly observed therapy). Twice-weekly and once-weekly regimens have been associated with a significant risk of treatment failure, TB relapse and development of acquired rifamycin drug resistance when used to treat HIV-infected individuals, especially with low blood CD4 counts (<100 cells/µL).

Rifampicin is a potent inducer of the hepatic enzyme system cytochrome P450 (CYP450). It has numerous drug–drug interactions with other agents. Of particular importance are those with cART, where subtherapeutic levels of these drugs can lead to treatment failure and HIV drug resistance. An alternative rifamycin with a less marked effect on CYP450 is rifabutin. Although more expensive than rifampicin, outcome and tolerability appear similar when either agent is used. Other anti-TB drugs do not significantly interact with antiretrovirals.

Effective cART improves host immunity with a 60–90% risk reduction in the development of active TB. Even with an undetectable HIV load and a good blood CD4 count response, individuals are still at a considerably greater risk of TB than the general population. It should also be noted that the beneficial effect of cART takes several months, and in TB endemic areas rates of TB may actually increase during the first 3 months of cART.

The optimal regimen for combined use of cART and anti-TB therapy remains unclear (Table 9.3). In many countries the choice of cART may reflect local availability rather than virological potency or potential drug–drug interactions, although it is hoped that this is now changing. Nucleoside reverse transcriptase inhibitors (NRTIs) can all be easily combined with rifamycin-containing anti-TB regimens. The potent induction of CYP450 by rifampicin produces subtherapeutic levels of protease inhibitors (PIs) even with ritonavir boosting, and this combination should be avoided (Table 9.4). Rifabutin is a useful alternative; however, most PIs inhibit rifabutin metabolism causing supranormal levels, and adverse effects of the rifamycin dose is not reduced. Hence careful, expert dose management is required.

The effect of rifampicin on nucleoside reverse transcriptase inhibitors (NNRTIs) is not as marked, and safe and effective co-administration of the NNRTI efavirenz is possible, although the dose may need to be increased in heavier subjects (weight >60 kg). Nevirapine is an alternative NNRTI that is frequently used

**Table 9.3** Current first-line UK cART regimens for use with antituberculosis therapy in subjects with no significant HIV drug resistance (Note: All other antituberculosis agents are safe to combine with cART without adjustment).

| cART regimen | Rifamycin dose | cART modification |
|---|---|---|
| Two nucleosides plus efavirenz | 1. Rifampicin 600 mg od | Efavirenz 600 mg od (increase to 800 mg if >60 kg) |
| | 2. Rifabutin 450 mg od | None required |
| Two nucleosides plus boosted protease inhibitor | Rifabutin 150 mg three times a week | None required |

**Table 9.4** Interaction between rifampicin or rifabutin (RBT) with protease inhibitors (PIs), non-nucleoside reverse transcriptase inhibitors (NNRTIs), integrase inhibitors and entry inhibitors.

| | Rifampicin | Rifabutin |
|---|---|---|
| **PI** | | |
| Unboosted PI | Do not use | Reduce RBT to 150 mg od* |
| Ritonavir boosted PI | Do not use | Reduce RBT to 150 mg thrice weekly |
| **NNRTI** | | |
| Efavirenz | See Table 9.3 | Increase RBT to 450 mg od |
| Nevirapine | Not recommended | Not recommended |
| Etravirine | Do not use | Not recommended |
| Rilpivirine | Do not use | Not recommended |
| **Integrase inhibitors** | | |
| Raltegravir | Not recommended | Standard drug doses |
| Elvitegravir | Do not use | Do not use |
| **Entry inhibitors** | | |
| Maraviroc | Not recommended | Standard doses |
| Enfuvirtide | Standard doses | Standard doses |

*Do not use with Indinavir or Saquinavir monotherapy.

in a fixed-dose generic cART regimen in resource-poor settings. Rifampicin reduces plasma nevirapine levels, and this combination should be used with caution even though the high therapeutic index for nevirapine may somewhat ameliorate this effect in clinical practice. As with much in this area, studies are awaited in patient cohorts treated under programmatic conditions in different parts of the world. The same applies to newer antiretroviral agents such as the fusion, integrase and co-receptor inhibitors, many of which require dose adjustment if being used during anti-TB treatment (Table 9.4).

It is generally agreed that effective TB treatment should be the first priority in an HIV-infected individual with active TB. The decision when to start cART in treatment-naïve subjects needs to balance the risk of progression to AIDS and death (if cART is deferred) with the potential for problems associated with concurrent (early) treatment. These include overlapping toxicities, increased pill burden and risk of suboptimal adherence, drug–drug interactions and inflammatory reactions (Box 9.1). The risks and benefits of cART are both most frequent during the first 2 months of anti-TB treatment – especially in patients who most need cART, i.e. with blood CD4 counts <100 cells/μL at baseline. Recent data have helped to clarify the optimal timing of cART initiation, and it is recommended that it is started as soon as practical in subjects with blood CD4 counts <350 cells/μL. In resource-rich environments this may be as long as several weeks to months if the blood CD4 count is >100 cells/μL, and *Pneumocystis* prophylaxis is used. Subjects with very low CD4 counts will usually be encouraged to start within 2 weeks of anti-TB treatment.

---

Box 9.1 **Starting cART in patients on TB treatment – risks of early and delayed therapy**

**Early (within 2 weeks) concomitant use**

- Risk of drug–drug interactions
- Overlapping toxicities and additive adverse effects
- High pill burden
- Risk of reduced patient adherence
- Immune reconstitution inflammatory syndrome

**Delay in concomitant use**

- Risk of other major opportunistic infections and death

---

Severe adverse events pose potential obstacles to the successful treatment of HIV and TB. They have been reported to occur almost twice as often in co-infected patients. Particular problems were seen in the past with drugs such as thiacetazone, which produced a high incidence of severe rash, and stavudine (peripheral neuropathy – in particular with isoniazid). Using modern rifamycin-based regimens the most commonly encountered severe adverse events are hepatotoxicity, peripheral neuropathy, rash and persistent nausea and vomiting. Some of these, such as neuropathy, may in fact be related predominantly to underlying HIV infection. The available evidence suggests that many adverse events can be managed without either cART or anti-TB therapy interruption. Nevertheless, care should be taken when considering the use of drug combinations with overlapping toxicities.

## Immune reconstitution inflammatory syndrome

Since the introduction of cART, HIV physicians have become aware of the potential for drug therapy to worsen existing disease or reveal new conditions as part of the immune reconstitution inflammatory syndrome (IRIS). This was recognized in HIV-negative individuals treated for TB many years ago and was termed a paradoxical reaction. cART use, particularly when introduced within a few weeks of starting TB treatment, appears to have increased the frequency and severity of these reactions two- to fivefold (consensus definition for paradoxical type IRIS, Box 9.2). The mechanism underlying this is unclear, but predisposing factors may include severely impaired baseline immunity (often expressed as very low blood CD4 counts), and disseminated TB (suggesting a large host mycobacterial burden) (Figure 9.4a,b).

---

Box 9.2 **Case definition for paradoxical tuberculosis-associated immune reconstitution inflammatory syndrome (IRIS)**

There are three components to the case definition:

**(A) Antecedent requirements**

Both of the two following requirements must be met:

- Diagnosis of tuberculosis: the tuberculosis diagnosis was made before starting cART and this should fulfil WHO criteria for diagnosis of smear-positive pulmonary tuberculosis, smear-negative pulmonary tuberculosis, or extrapulmonary tuberculosis
- Initial response to tuberculosis treatment: the patient's condition should have stabilized or improved on appropriate tuberculosis treatment before cART initiation, e.g. cessation of night sweats, fevers, cough, weight loss. (Note: this does not apply to patients starting cART within 2 weeks of commencing tuberculosis treatment as insufficient time may have elapsed for a clinical response to be reported)

**(B) Clinical criteria**

The onset of tuberculosis-associated IRIS manifestations should be within 3 months of cART initiation, re-initiation or regimen change because of treatment failure.

Of the following, at least one major criterion or two minor clinical criteria are required:

**Major criteria**

- New or enlarging lymph nodes, cold abscesses, or other focal tissue involvement – e.g. tuberculous arthritis
- New or worsening radiological features of tuberculosis (found by chest radiography, abdominal ultrasonography, CT or MRI)
- New or worsening CNS tuberculosis (meningitis or focal neurological deficit – e.g. caused by tuberculoma)
- New or worsening serositis (pleural effusion, ascites or pericardial effusion)

**Minor criteria**

- New or worsening constitutional symptoms such as fever, night sweats or weight loss

- New or worsening respiratory symptoms such as cough, dyspnoea or stridor
- New or worsening abdominal pain accompanied by peritonitis, hepatomegaly, splenomegaly or abdominal adenopathy

**(C) Alternative explanations for clinical deterioration must be excluded if possible**

- Failure of tuberculosis treatment because of tuberculosis drug resistance
- Poor adherence to tuberculosis treatment
- Another opportunistic infection or neoplasm (particularly important in patients with smear-negative pulmonary tuberculosis and extrapulmonary tuberculosis where the initial tuberculosis diagnosis has not been confirmed microbiologically)
- Drug toxicity or reaction

*Source:* Adapted from Meintjes G. *Lancet Infect Dis* 2008;8:516

---

Reported manifestations of IRIS are numerous and may mimic adverse drug reactions, progressive disease due to resistance, inadequate drug levels because of malabsorption, drug–drug interactions or non-adherence, or the presence of an alternative diagnosis such as lymphoma or another infection. IRIS can also occur in an 'unmasking form', where subjects who are not known to have active TB develop an acute, inflammatory form of TB within a few weeks of starting cART. The precise incidence of this form of disease is unknown, but in its most severe form is likely to be relatively infrequent.

There is currently no specific test for IRIS, and it should always be regarded as a diagnosis of exclusion following assessment for the conditions listed above. Generally it can be managed without interruption of either anti TB therapy or cART. Less severe cases will often resolve without additional therapy. However, more serious or prolonged events, especially when associated with worsening cerebral or mediastinal disease likely to cause compression of vital structures, should be treated with systemic corticosteroids. The patient needs to be monitored carefully for response as well as adverse effects of steroid therapy, which include hyperglycaemia, hypertension, bone demineralization and reactivation of local and systemic viral infections.

## TB control

Although prior to HIV high TB burden countries focused on detection and treatment of infectious cases of active TB, it is now appreciated that optimal TB control requires LTBI management plus exclusion of subclinical TB. Like most aspects of TB/HIV, this is not without complication. For example, interpretation of the standard diagnostics in LTBI (tuberculin skin test and blood interferon gamma release assays) becomes more problematic as an individual's blood CD4 count falls. However, our understanding of the interaction between TB and HIV is considerably better than it was just 5 years ago, and we have better rapid diagnostic tests available for active disease plus novel anti-TB agents that may enable therapeutic duration to be considerably shortened for both latent and active TB treatments.

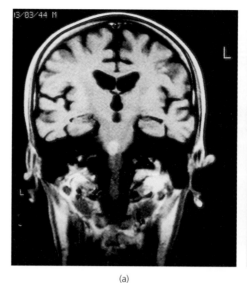 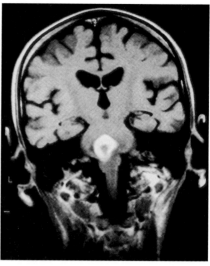

(a)                                    (b)

**Figure 9.4** (a) MR image showing a mid-brain tuberculosis mass lesion with gadolinium enhancement prior to starting cART. (b) MR image of same patient 2 weeks after starting cART. There is now increased gadolinium enhancement associated with new neurological signs.

Irrespective of geographic setting, TB control is limited without adequate HIV control. Policies such as the WHO Directly Observed Therapy Short course (DOTS) strategy (Box 9.3) should incorporate both HIV testing and treatment programmes. To be effective these must be integrated and implemented at local and national levels and come with clear political backing. Sadly, in some parts of the world, this remains far from ideal.

---

Box 9.3 **Fundamental elements of the WHO DOTS strategy**

**1** Political commitment with increased and sustained finance by national Governments
**2** Case-detection through quality assured bacteriology services
**3** Standardized treatment with supervision (DOTS) and patient support
**4** An effective drug supply and management system
**5** A system to monitor and evaluate the effect of the strategy

*Source:* Adapted from www.who.int/tb/dots/whatisdots/en/index.html.

---

## Further reading

British HIV Association. Guidelines for the Treatment of TB/HIV Coinfection 2011. (http://www.bhiva.org/TB-HIV2011.aspx).

Dye C, Williams BG. The population dynamics and control of tuberculosis. *Science* 2010;328:856–861.

Lawn SD, Török ME, Wood R. Optimum time to start antiretroviral therapy during HIV-associated opportunistic infections. *Curr Opin Infect Dis* 2011;24:34–42.

Lipman M, Breen R. Immune reconstitution inflammatory syndrome in HIV. *Curr Opin Infect Dis* 2006;19:20–25.

Martinson NA, Hoffmann CJ, Chaisson RE. Epidemiology of tuberculosis and HIV: recent advances in understanding and responses. *Proc Am Thorac Soc* 2011;8:288–293.

Pozniak A, Coyne K, Miller R, *et al.* on behalf of the BHIVA Guidelines Subcommittee. *HIV Med* 2011;12:517–524.

# CHAPTER 10

# The Gut and HIV

*B. Gazzard[1] and M. Nelson[2]*

[1]Imperial College London, London, UK
[2]Chelsea and Westminster Hospital, London, UK

## OVERVIEW

- In the pre-cART era infections and tumours of the gastrointestinal tract were common
- With the advent of successful therapy these have become less prevalent and the commonest gastrointestinal (GI) symptom is diarrhoea as a side effect from antiretroviral medication
- Individuals unaware of their HIV diagnosis may present with GI symptoms and consideration of HIV testing should be considered if symptoms remain unexplained
- In the HIV population many abdominal symptoms may be related to non-HIV-associated causes and referral to an experienced gastroenterologist may be needed

## Introduction

The gastrointestinal tract can be affected at all stages of HIV infection and symptoms related to the gut are the most frequent in individuals living with HIV. Prior to the introduction of combination antiretroviral therapy (cART), the majority of these symptoms were associated with opportunistic infections and HIV-related tumours. However, with the success of cART the majority of gastrointestinal disease is now aetiologically similar to that of the HIV-negative population except for toxicities related to antiretroviral agents. It is important, however, that all physicians are aware of the possible manifestations of HIV-associated disease of the gastrointestinal tract as these may be the first clinical manifestation of symptomatic HIV disease and should prompt the clinician to offer HIV testing. Additionally, gastrointestinal (GI) problems can occur in individuals taking cART if there is lack of HIV virological control or persistent immunosuppression.

In patients with HIV infection, the risk and pattern of GI involvement alter with the level of immune function, and in particular with the CD4 count. Whereas some are AIDS-defining conditions (Box 10.1) others may occur at any stage of HIV disease. The gut mucosa is an important route of entry of HIV and in those practicing anal intercourse it is important to exclude other sexually acquired infections which may affect the lower gastrointestinal tract.

*ABC of HIV and AIDS*, Sixth Edition. Edited by Michael W. Adler,
Simon G. Edwards, Robert F. Miller, Gulshan Sethi and Ian G. Williams.
© 2012 Blackwell Publishing Ltd. Published 2012 by Blackwell Publishing Ltd.

Box 10.1 **AIDS defining conditions affecting the GI tract**

**Infections**

- Oesophogeal candidiasis
- Cytomegalovirus (other than liver, spleen and lymph nodes)
- Cryptosporidiosis for greater than 1 month
- Chronic herpes simplex infection for greater than 1 month
- Chronic isosporiosis for greater than 1 month
- *Mycobacterium tuberculosis* infection
- *Mycobacterium avium-intracellulare* infection
- Recurrent salmonella septicaemia

**Tumours**

- Kaposi sarcoma
- Burkitt's lymphoma
- Immunoblastic lymphoma

## Dysphagia and odynophagia

Dysphagia (difficulty swallowing) and odynophagia (pain on swallowing) are common symptoms in those with late stage untreated HIV disease, but these symptoms may occur at any stage of HIV infection. HIV seroconversion may occasionally be complicated by aphthous ulceration of the oesophagus with the development of these symptoms, but generally more classical symptoms of seroconversion will also be present.

The commonest cause of dysphagia and odynophagia in HIV disease is oesophageal candidiasis. In the majority of cases plaques of candida are also present in the mouth (Figure 10.1) and the diagnosis can be inferred, with symptoms usually resolving following antifungal therapy. Where the diagnosis is in doubt or symptoms do not resolve with treatment an endoscopy should be performed where the appearances of oesophageal candida are typical (Figure 10.2) and can be confirmed by brushings or histology. Standard treatment for oesophageal candida is with an azole most commonly fluconazole. Occasionally candida species may be resistant to fluconazole and may respond to itraconazole. In those unable to swallow, intravenous therapy with amphotericin B or caspofungin is required.

A minority of HIV positive individuals with oesophageal symptoms have other opportunistic infections. Herpes simplex (HSV) infection and cytomegalovirus (CMV) may both produce distal

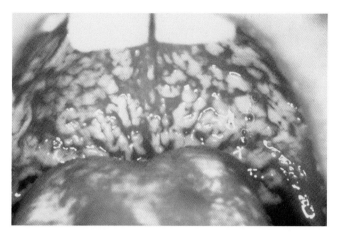

**Figure 10.1** Oral candida.

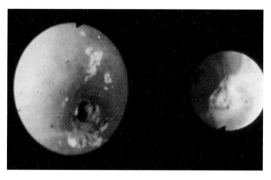

**Figure 10.3** Cytomegalovirus affecting the oesophagus: endoscopic appearance demonstrating ulceration in oesophagus.

oesophagitis and typically occur at CD4 counts below 100 cells/μL, and often co-exist with candidiasis. CMV is associated with discrete ulceration with rolled edges resembling a carcinoma (Figure 10.3). CMV oesophagitis is treated with ganciclovir intravenously, and HSV oesophagitis by intravenous aciclovir. All patients with CMV oesophagitis should be screened for retinal disease. Apthous ulceration of the oesophagus may be due to an unknown virus or HIV itself and usually responds to Thalidomide or intralesional or systemic steroids. Kaposi sarcoma (KS), and more rarely lymphoma, may affect the oesophagus.

## Nausea and vomiting

In the pre-cART era nausea and vomiting were primarily associated with opportunistic infections most commonly those that cause HIV diarrhoea (Table 10.1) and tumours, both KS and lymphoma, of the stomach. Nowadays they are most commonly associated with cART especially, but not exclusively, with ritonavir-boosted protease inhibitors. Nausea and vomiting are linked to non-adherence to cART regimens and should be actively treated. The possibility of these symptoms being secondary to HIV related CNS infection or tumours should always be considered.

## Diarrhoea

Prior to the introduction of cART it was estimated that 30–70% of individuals experienced diarrhoea, which was primarily linked to infections (Table 10.1) and tumours. cART has greatly reduced the prevalence, although diarrhoea may be a common side effect of cART itself. All individuals experiencing diarrhoea should have stool cultures sent, and if no cause is found and the diarrhoea continues should be referred for further investigation, which most commonly would include sigmoidoscopy/colonoscopy and possibly upper gastrointestinal endoscopy.

### Acute diarrhoea

Patients presenting with a sudden onset of diarrhoea may have any of the causes of chronic diarrhoea (see below) but are more likely to have either a bacterial or viral infection.

### Bacterial infections

*Salmonella, Shigella* and *Campylobacter* are enteropathogens which occur with increased frequency in HIV-infected individuals. The illness is usually more severe than in the immunocompetent, is more likely to relapse and infections are caused by less virulent species. *Salmonella* and *Campylobacter* are associated with food contamination and are prevented by good food hygiene and thorough cooking. *Shigella* infection is both water-borne and sexually

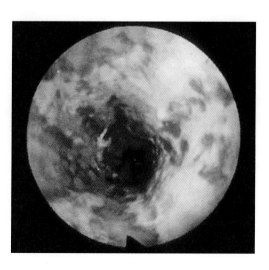

**Figure 10.2** Fibreoptic appearances of oesophageal candida.

**Table 10.1**   Major causes of HIV-related diarrhoea

| Bacteria | Parasites | Viruses | Non-infectious |
|---|---|---|---|
| Campylobacter spp | *Cryptosporidium* spp | Cytomegalovirus | Combined antiretroviral therapy |
| *Clostridium difficile* | *Cyclospora cayetanensis* | Herpes simplex viruses | |
| *Escherichia coli* Salmonella spp | *Giardia lamblia* Entamoeba histolytica Isospora belli Strongyloides stercoralis | Rotavirus Norovirus | |
| Shigella spp | | | Lymphoma: Hodgkin and non-Hodgkin |
| *Mycobacterium tuberculosis* | | | |
| *Mycobacterium avium-intracellulare* complex | | | |
| *Mycobacterium kansasii* | | | |

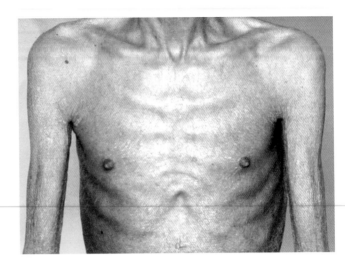

**Figure 10.4** HIV wasting syndrome.

transmitted, but is comparatively rare. All three organisms respond to ciprofloxacin, although there are increasing reports of resistance. *Clostridium difficile* is an important cause of diarrhoea and is more common in the severely immunosuppressed but the presenting symptoms are similar. Treatment is similar to that in the seronegative population. Sexually transmitted agents including *Neisseria gonorrhoeae* and *Chlamydia* species, especially *Lymphogranuloma venereum* should always be considered.

## Viral infections

Acute diarrhoea may be caused by rotavirus or very occasionally adenovirus which when it does occur may cause a protracted illness with no known treatment. Herpes simplex infection may present with a severe proctocolitis and acute diarrhoea.

## Chronic diarrhoea

In the pre-cART era chronic diarrhoea was common and was an important contributor to the wasting syndrome (Figure 10.4).

The necessary investigations and the likely causes of chronic diarrhoea vary depending upon the degree of immunosuppression as assessed by the CD4 count. With a count of above 200 cells/μL opportunistic infections are unlikely and investigation should be similar to that in general gastroenterology, with the irritable bowel syndrome being the commonest diagnosis.

In those with a CD4 count below 200 cells/μL it is important that HIV-related infections and tumours are always excluded. Possible infectious causes are discussed below.

## Microsporidium

These are obligate intracellular parasites that occur most commonly in those with a CD4 count below 100 cells/μL. The most common species causing gastrointestinal disease are *Enterocytozoon bieneusi* and *Septata intestinalis*, the latter also being associated with renal and corneal damage.

Microsporidial cysts are ingested from contaminated water and in the alkaline pH of the duodenal fluid cysts extrude a thin tube which penetrates the duodenal mucosa like a hypodermic needle and the contents of the cyst are injected into the cell (Figure 10.5). Infection usually produces mild to moderate watery, non-bloody diarrhoea. Stool examination with specific fluorescent stains is usually sufficient for diagnosis (see Figure 10.6) but if stool specimens are negative a small bowel biopsy may be required for diagnosis.

Asymptomatic infections rarely occur and like cryptosporidium, microsporidial infection may resolve spontaneously in those with better preserved CD4 counts. *Septata intestinalis* can be eradicated by albendazole but there is no treatment for *Enterocytozoon bieneusi*. Successful treatment with cART due to improvement of immune function, leads to eradication of microsporidia with resolution of symptoms.

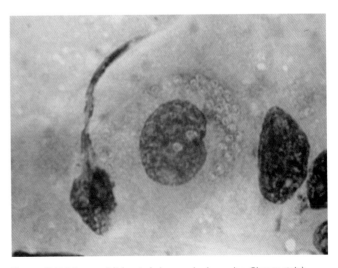

**Figure 10.5** Microsporidial cysts (microscopic view using Giemsa stain) (courtesy of Elizabeth Canning).

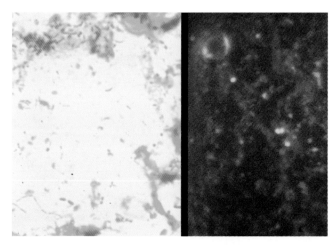

**Figure 10.6** Microscopic stool examination using fluorescent stain showing microsporidial cysts.

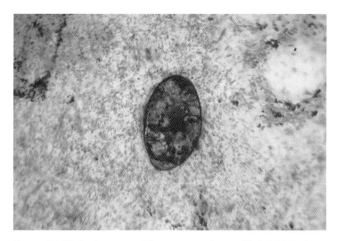

**Figure 10.7** Stained cryptosporidium oocysts using modified Ziehl–Neelsen stain.

## Cryptosporidium

This is a protozoa that commonly infects the immunocompetent producing acute attacks of diarrhoea. However, in the immunosupressed, particularly those with a CD4 count less than 100 cells/µL, it may cause severe chronic diarrhoea often associated with nausea, malabsorption and anorexia leading to rapid and extensive weight loss. The stool volumes in cryptosporidial diarrhoea are variable but in some patients more than 1 L of stool is passed daily. The commonest source is contaminated water and this infection can be prevented by boiling water to destroy cryptosporidial cysts. Diagnosis is by stool examination with auramine and acid fast stains (Figure 10.7). Diagnosis may also be achieved by obtaining colonic or rectal biopsy which may demonstrate oocysts attached to the epithelial cells (Figure 10.8). No treatment has been shown to eradicate cryptosporidium reliably, although paromomycin and nitazoxanide may be utilized. The best therapy once more is cART with restoration of the immune system again leading to eradication and resolution of symptoms.

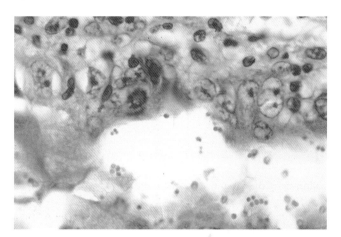

**Figure 10.8** Rectal biopsy showing cryptosprodialoocysts attached to the epithelial cells.

## Cytomegalovirus colitis

Although cytomegalovirus (CMV) infection may occur throughout the gastrointestinal tract, CMV colitis is its most common manifestation occurring most commonly in those with a CD4 count below 50 cells/µL. Disease follows reactivation of a previous CMV infection, which is common in the HIV infected population. Classically, patients present with bloody diarrhoea, and the macroscopic appearance at endoscopy is typical of a colitis (Figure 10.9). The diagnosis is confirmed by finding typical viral inclusions on histology of colonic biopsies (Figure 10.10). Complications of perforation or toxic dilatation may occur in a small number of patients. Treatment is with either foscarnet or ganciclovir and relapses are prevented by initiation of successful cART. Active retinal infection must be excluded in all those diagnosed with CMV colitis.

## Other infections

Other infections associated with chronic diarrhoea include *Giardia*, which commonly has associated symptoms of nausea, bloating

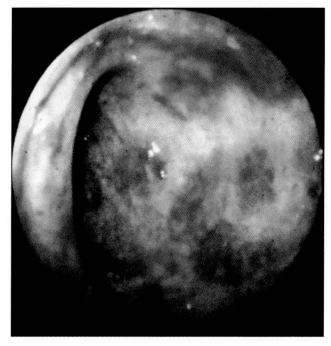

**Figure 10.9** Cytomegalovirus colitis: macroscopic appearance at endoscopy.

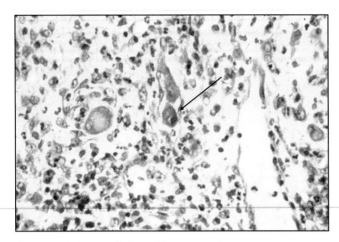

**Figure 10.10** Cytomegalovirus colitis: macroscopic appearance at endoscopy.

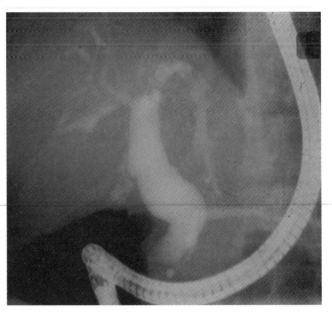

**Figure 10.11** AIDS-related sclerosing cholangitis: ERCP image shows typical beaded appearance of the intra- and extrahepatic ducts.

and chronic abdominal pain; *Entaemoeba histolytica*, which may present with fever, bloody or watery diarrhoea and abdominal pain; *Cyclospora* associated with prolonged watery diarrhoea; *Isospora belli* and *Strongyloides*. Diagnosis is through stool specimen with specific staining and occasionally colonic biopsy is required.

### Tumours

Both KS and HIV-associated lymphoma may occur in the lower gastrointestinal tract and be associated with diarrhoea. Colonic cancer may be commoner than the general population in those who are HIV infected and over the age of 50.

### Drugs

In the cART era perhaps the commonest reversible cause of diarrhoea is drug therapy with non-HIV agents, although it is particularly associated with antiretroviral agents especially ritonavir boosted protease inhibitors. With a now widely available choice of HIV drugs, switching either within class or to a different class of agent will often lead to resolution.

### Other causes

With success of HIV therapy leading to a reduction in opportunistic infections and HIV-associated tumours, non-HIV-associated conditions should always be considered. When there is difficulty making a diagnosis referral to an experienced gastroenterologist is essential. Some conditions associated with diarrhoea may occur more frequently in the HIV population, e.g. malabsorption secondary to exocrine pancreatic insufficiency and may be the consequence of long-term antiretroviral exposure.

### Abdominal pain

Abdominal pain is common in the general population and is similarly so in those infected with HIV. Although abdominal pain may have myriad causes both in and outside of the gastrointestinal tract, there are some specific HIV-related diagnoses that must be kept in mind.

### Right upper quadrant pain

Right upper quadrant pain may be associated with AIDS-related sclerosing cholangitis (Figure 10.11). This condition is pathologically and radiologically identical to idiopathic sclerosing cholangitis with irregular dilatation and narrowing of both the intrahepatic and extrahepatic ducts caused by areas of fibrosis. The condition occurs predominantly in those with a CD4 count less than 100 cells/μL. Virtually all cases of AIDS-related sclerosing cholangitis are associated with microsporidium, cryptosporidium or cytomegalovirus infection, and diarrhoea is thus a common accompaniment. Very severe pain is associated with papillary stenosis. As cART is associated with the eradication of the opportunistic infections leading to this condition, it is now rare. Acute acalculous cholecystitis may be commoner than in the general population especially in late stage HIV infection.

### Acute appendicitis

Appendicitis may be commoner in HIV-positive patients, probably due to an association with cytomegalovirus infection.

### Acute pancreatitis

Acute pancreatitis may be associated with infections including cytomegalovirus. The commonest cause however is antiviral therapy particularly didanosine. Severe hypertriglyceridaemia associated with cART may also be an associated causative factor.

### Generalized abdominal pain

The commonest cause for generalized abdominal pain is severe constipation associated with opiate use. Cytomegalovirus infection may present with severe abdominal pain and rebound tenderness and diarrhoea. *Mycobacterium avium-intracellulare* (MAI) classically presents with severe abdominal pain, a raised alkaline phosphatase, anaemia and fever. The abdominal pain is sometimes associated with massive enlargement of the intra-abdominal lymph nodes. Treatment with corticosteroids may produce short-term palliation of the pain and specific anti-MAI therapy should be introduced, although the development of resistance is common. Successful cART treatment is associated with eradication of the organism. Lymph node enlargement secondary to lymphoma may also present in this way.

## Anal pain

Anal pain may be secondary to infection from herpes simplex infection or in those with a low CD4 count CMV infection. Other sexually acquired conditions particularly *Lymphogranuloma venereum* may present with perianal pain commonly associated with a bloody mucus discharge. Perianal abscesses and fissures are relatively common. Carcinoma of the anus (see Figure 7.11) occurs more commonly in men who have sex with men and the HIV population in general.

## Further reading

British HIV Association. Guidelines Writing Group on Opportunistic Infection. *HIV Med* 2011;12(Suppl 2):1468–1293.

Nelson MR, Shanson DC, Hawkins DA, Gazzard BG. Salmonella, Campylobacter and Shigella in HIV-seropositive patients. *AIDS* 1992;6:1495–1498.

Ng SC, Gazzard B. Advances in sexually transmitted infections of the gastrointestinal tract. *Nat Rev Gastroenterol Hepatol* 2009;6:592–607.

Shacklett BL, Anton PA. HIV Infection and gut mucosal immune function: updates on pathogenesis with implications for management and intervention. *Curr Infect Dis Rep* 2010;12:19–27.

# CHAPTER 11

# Viral Hepatitis and Liver Disease

*R. Gilson and H. Price*

University College London, London, UK

**OVERVIEW**

- End-stage chronic liver disease and hepatocellular carcinoma cause an increasing proportion of deaths in HIV-positive individuals
- The major underlying cause is viral hepatitis co-infection, either hepatitis B or hepatitis C, although antiretrovirals themselves can cause major hepatotoxicity
- HIV-positive persons are now considered as potential transplant candidates since the improvement in the prognosis of the underlying HIV disease
- There is an epidemic of sexually transmitted hepatitis C among HIV-infected men who have sex with men
- Prevention is key. All HIV-infected individuals should be immunized against hepatitis A and B

## Introduction

The liver is not directly affected by HIV infection itself; however, end-stage chronic liver disease and hepatocellular carcinoma cause an increasing proportion of deaths in HIV-positive individuals. The major underlying cause is viral hepatitis co-infection, either hepatitis B virus (HBV) or hepatitis C virus (HCV). In patients with a history of injecting drug use or blood product exposure, HCV is the most common; in other groups it is HBV.

All newly diagnosed HIV-positive patients should be tested for hepatitis virus infection (Tables 11.1–11.4), as part of a baseline assessment for liver disease (Box 11.1). If not immune, patients should be given hepatitis A and hepatitis B vaccines. Both vaccines are safe in HIV-positive patients, although the antibody response rates are lower, particularly for hepatitis B vaccine, where only 50% patients develop a strong antibody response (at least 100 IU/L anti-HBs) (Box 11.2).

Box 11.1 **Assessment of the newly diagnosed HIV-positive patient**

- History
  - blood or blood product exposure
  - injecting drug use
  - alcohol intake
- Investigation
  - liver function tests
  - serology for hepatitis A, B and C

Box 11.2 **Hepatitis vaccination in the HIV-positive patient**

- Hepatitis A and B vaccination recommended, if not previously exposed
- No safety issues
- Standard doses/schedule
- Reduced seroconversion rate, particularly for hepatitis B, related to CD4 count
- Hepatitis B vaccine: up to 3 further doses for poor or non-responders to a first course
- Booster dose recommended when anti-HBs level drops below 100 IU/L

**Table 11.1** Indications for use of hepatitis B marker tests.

| Clinical scenario | HBsAg | Anti-HBs | Anti-HBc | HBeAg | Anti-HBe | HBV DNA | Comments |
|---|---|---|---|---|---|---|---|
| Newly diagnosed HIV | ✓ | ✓ | ✓ | | | | Screen for current or past infection |
| Post-vaccine follow-up | | ✓ | | | | | Vaccinate only if initial screen negative |
| If HBsAg positive | ✓ | | | ✓ | ✓ | ✓ | Repeat annually |
| If cleared infection | ✓ | | | | | | To detect reactivation |

*ABC of HIV and AIDS*, Sixth Edition. Edited by Michael W. Adler, Simon G. Edwards, Robert F. Miller, Gulshan Sethi and Ian G. Williams.
© 2012 Blackwell Publishing Ltd. Published 2012 by Blackwell Publishing Ltd.

## Hepatitis B co-infection

Hepatitis B co-infection is frequent because of the common routes of infection and risk factors. In areas where hepatitis B is endemic

**Table 11.2** Indications for use of hepatitis C tests.

| Clinical scenario | Anti-HCV | HCV RNA | Comments |
|---|---|---|---|
| Newly diagnosed HIV | ✓ | | Repeat annually if initially negative |
| If anti-HCV positive | | ✓ | To distinguish current and past infection or detect reinfection |

**Table 11.3** Tests for hepatitis B, and their interpretation.

| | HBsAg | Anti-HBs | Anti-HBc | Anti-HBc IgM | HBeAg | Anti-HBe | HBV DNA |
|---|---|---|---|---|---|---|---|
| Never infected | − | − | − | | | | |
| Immune following a course of vaccine | − | + | − | | | | |
| Immune following a natural infection | − | + | + | | | | |
| Acute infection: | | | | | | | |
| Early/pre-symptomatic | + | − | − | − | +/− | − | |
| Late/symptomatic | + | − | + | ++ | + | − | |
| Chronic infection: | | | | | | | |
| • high infectivity | + | − | + | +/− | + | − | ++ |
| • low infectivity | + | − | + | − | − | + | + |

in the general population, most infections are acquired by mother to child or early childhood infection. Infections acquired at this age persist (chronic infection) in 80–90% cases. Consequently co-infection rates are high in individuals who are subsequently at risk of acquiring HIV infection. This is typical of the situation in

**Table 11.4** Tests for hepatitis C, and their interpretation.

| | Anti-HCV | HCV RNA |
|---|---|---|
| Never infected | − | − |
| Past infection | + | − |
| Acute infection | − | + |
| Chronic infection | + | + |

much of sub-Saharan Africa where hepatitis B carrier rates in the general population are in the range of 5–10% (Figure 11.1).

In regions such as Europe and North America, the carrier rate in the general population is much lower (as low as 0.1% in the UK). Here most infections are acquired as adults, or adolescents, related to behavioural risks, principally sexual behaviour or injecting drug use. Among HIV-positive patients, 40–60% have serological markers of hepatitis B infection, and 5% are co-infected with chronic hepatitis B.

## Acute hepatitis B

Clinical presentation is unaffected by HIV infection. However hepatitis B virus infection is more likely to follow a chronic course, affecting 20% of adult cases (compared to less than 5% in HIV-negative individuals).

## Chronic hepatitis B

Patients with chronic hepatitis B (HBsAg still detectable after 6 months) are all initially HBeAg positive with a high level of hepatitis B viral load (HBV DNA) and often normal liver function tests. This immune-tolerant phase is characterized by weak or undetectable HBV-specific T-cell immune responses. After months to years, most individuals will develop stronger multispecific immune responses, increased liver disease activity, raised transaminase levels,

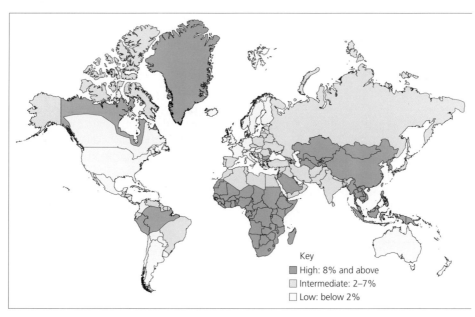

Key
■ High: 8% and above
▢ Intermediate: 2–7%
□ Low: below 2%

**Figure 11.1** World map showing prevalence of hepatitis B virus infection as defined by WHO. *Source:* Gill G. & Beeching N. *Lecture Notes Tropical Medicine 6e*. Reproduced with permission of John Wiley & Sons, Ltd.

and go on to control HBV replication with a fall in HBV viral load and seroconversion from HBeAg to anti-HBe. This stage is delayed or prevented in HIV-positive patients, such that the rate of spontaneous HBeAg to anti-HBe seroconversion is reduced from 10% to 5% per year.

In patients who remain HBeAg negative with low HBV viral load of less than 20 000 IU/mL ($10^5$ copies/mL), most have normal or near normal (<1.5 times the upper limit of normal) alanine aminotransferase (ALT) and a low risk of progression of liver disease. However, HIV infection increases the risk of progression of liver disease in this group and the risk of reactivation of viral replication with a switch back to HBeAg positivity. Consequently, the overall risk of developing end-stage liver disease is increased.

## Treatment of chronic hepatitis B

Any patient with chronic hepatitis B is a potential candidate for treatment to prevent liver disease progression. The indications for treatment in HIV co-infection are the same as for HIV-negative patients. The viral load threshold for considering treatment is 2000 IU/mL, reflecting the increased risk of progression. UK guidelines recommend long-term antiviral therapy with the aim of maintaining sustained suppression of viral replication (undetectable HBV viral load). If a patient needs to start treatment for their HBV infection, they should consider starting combination antiretroviral therapy (cART) with a regimen including drugs active against both HIV and HBV, even if their CD4 count is above the threshold where cART would usually be recommended. For patients who do not want to start cART the options are limited to adefovir with or without telbivudine, or a course of pegylated interferon, if genotype A.

All patients with hepatitis B should be tested for hepatitis delta virus because, if positive, it may be an indication for earlier treatment.

## Hepatitis C co-infection

Most cases of hepatitis C are diagnosed as a result of screening or investigation of abnormal liver function tests. Overall, the prevalence of co-infection in the UK is about 9%, but the prevalence varies markedly by risk group (Table 11.5).

## Acute hepatitis C

There is an epidemic of acute hepatitis C among HIV-positive men who have sex with men (MSM). It is thought the route of transmission is unprotected anal sex. Injecting drug users are also at

**Table 11.5** Prevalence of hepatitis C co-infection by risk group in the UK.

| Risk category | HCV antibody positive (%) |
|---|---|
| MSM | 7.2 |
| IDU | 83.7 |
| Heterosexual | 4.4 |
| Unknown/other | 8.3 |

IDU, injecting drug user; MSM, men who have sex with men.

risk. All HIV-positive individuals should be screened for hepatitis C annually with more frequent testing considered in those at greatest risk. Only 10% of acute hepatitis C infections are symptomatic. As with hepatitis B, the proportion of HCV infections that persist is higher in HIV-positive patients. Less than 10% clear infection within 6 months, compared with 20–30% in HIV-negative patients. Most acute HCV infections in HIV-positive patients are detected through routine liver function test monitoring (usually just a raised ALT/AST (aspartate aminotransferase)). Treatment with pegylated interferon and ribavirin initiated within 6–12 months of seroconversion is probably more effective than if given later, but has not been subjected to a randomized trial.

## Natural history of chronic hepatitis C

There is strong evidence for a faster rate of progression of liver disease in HIV-co-infected patients with hepatitis C, with an estimated median time to cirrhosis of 15 years compared with 20–25 years in HIV-negative patients. Cirrhotic patients, as in those with hepatitis monoinfections, are at risk of liver failure and hepatocellular carcinoma. It is recommended that HCV treatment should be considered in all patients and that cART should be started earlier than in non-co-infected patients.

## Treatment for chronic hepatitis C

Standard treatment for hepatitis C is with subcutaneous pegylated interferon (weekly) and oral ribavirin (twice daily). Either interferon-α2a (Pegasys, Roche) or interferon-α2b (Viraferon Peg, Schering Plough) can be used; the dosages of the interferons differ, but both should be used with ribavirin at a dose adjusted for weight. Patients who are co-infected are more likely to require haemopoietic support with erythropoietin or granulocyte colony-stimulating factor if they are to avoid the need for dose reduction of ribavirin or interferon. Lower ribavirin doses are associated with a lower response rate, so should be avoided if possible. The absolute CD4 count falls with treatment, but the CD4% is usually maintained and therefore further action is rarely required. Treatment is otherwise the same as for HIV-negative patients; however, the response rates are lower. The response is about 50% in genotype 2 and 3 infection (compared with 75–80% in HIV-negative patients) and 20–30% in others (compared with 30–50%). In addition to genotype, the response to therapy at 4 and 12 weeks is predictive of the outcome. In patients who have not achieved an undetectable HCV viral load, or a >2 log fall from baseline, by week 12, therapy should be discontinued.

Apart from the limited efficacy, the major limitations of current treatment for hepatitis C are the side-effects of the treatment, which make it difficult to tolerate for many patients, and mean that they need specialist support (Box 11.3). New hepatitis C antiviral agents as adjuncts to interferon/ribavirin offer the prospect of improved response rates.

Didanosine is contraindicated in combination with ribavirin due to a drug interaction and abacavir may lower the response rate. Zidovudine is associated with an increased risk of anaemia.

Box 11.3 **Adverse effects of interferon/ribavirin therapy**

- Flu-like symptoms (fatigue, joint/muscle aches, fever, chills, headache)
- Haematological
  - Anaemia
  - Neutropenia
  - Thrombocytopenia
  - Decline in absolute CD4 count
- Neuropsychological
  - Depression
  - Irritability
  - Insomnia
- Dermatological
  - Injection site reactions
  - Dry skin
  - Itch
  - Alopecia
- Gastrointestinal
  - Nausea
  - Anorexia/weight loss
  - Pancreatitis
- Respiratory
  - Shortness of breath
  - Cough
- Metabolic
  - Lactic acidosis
- Retinopathy
- Teratogenicity

## Immune reconstitution

Recovery of immune responses to hepatitis virus infection, following initiation of cART, may lead to liver inflammation characterized by a 'flare' in the liver transaminase levels, and very rarely to liver decompensation in those with more severe chronic liver disease.

This is best described in hepatitis B in which recovery of HBV-specific CD8-positive lymphocyte responses leads to liver cell damage, largely mediated by non-specific cytotoxicity. This may be associated with a fall in hepatitis B viral load and occurs more often, but not exclusively, in patients starting antiretroviral regimens that include agents active against hepatitis B virus (lamivudine, emtricitabine or tenofovir). Although this is the characteristic pattern, there is no pathognomonic feature or diagnostic test to establish this as the cause of a flare. A similar pattern may also occur in patients with hepatitis C but is less frequent, and the immune mechanism is less well defined.

## Liver disease in an HIV-infected patient

Mild abnormalities of liver function tests, usually a raised ALT/AST up to twice the upper limit of normal are common in HIV infection.

**Table 11.6** Causes of liver disease in an HIV-infected patient.

| | |
|---|---|
| Hepatitis A | Acute hepatitis only |
| Hepatitis B | Acute or chronic hepatitis |
| Hepatitis C | Acute hepatitis uncommon; main cause of chronic hepatitis in IDU |
| Opportunistic Infections | TB, atypical mycobacteria, cryptococcosis, cytomegalovirus, microsporidiosis |
| Other infections | Syphilis |
| Tumours | Lymphoma, hepatocellular carcinoma |
| Metabolic | Steatohepatitis as part of the metabolic syndrome |
| Biliary | Sclerosing cholangitis, cryptosporidiosis |
| Drugs and alcohol | Includes self-medication with anabolic steroids |
| Antiretroviral drugs | All drugs potentially implicated, but particularly nevirapine and ritonavir* |
| Other conditions | Multicentric Castleman's disease |

*When ritonavir given as treatment dose i.e. 600 mg bd.

If not already known, it is essential to establish the viral hepatitis status of the patient and to consider alcohol and drug toxicity. Further investigation may not then be warranted as such abnormalities are often transient or intermittent. However, if the abnormality persists, or there are other symptoms that are not accounted for, and in all cases of jaundice, further investigation is required. Jaundice is never due to HIV infection alone. The main causes of acute and chronic liver disease in an HIV infected patient are shown in Table 11.6.

### cART and liver toxicity

A common management problem in HIV patients is deciding whether the development of abnormal liver function tests is an adverse reaction to cART.

Some antiretroviral drugs have clearly been associated with the development of hepatotoxicity, but all may have the potential to cause liver injury. Moderate elevations of ALT/AST (typically up to five times the upper limit of normal) usually resolve spontaneously, but any patient who becomes jaundiced or otherwise symptomatic or has ALT/AST >10 times the upper limit of normal should stop treatment immediately. Some changes may be misinterpreted as hepatotoxicity. Atazanavir, causes unconjugated hyperbilirubinaemia, and drugs such as nevirapine and efavirenz cause a rise in gamma glutamyl transferase due to enzyme induction. Patients with underlying liver disease, including asymptomatic carriers of hepatitis B or C, are at increased risk of clinically significant hepatotoxicity.

Most drug toxicity related to cART is not dose-dependent, or predictable. Hepatotoxicity may be a feature of hypersensitivity reactions associated with nevirapine, abacavir and protease inhibitors. This occurs typically soon after starting treatment (within a few days but up to 8 weeks).

Drugs that cause mitochondrial toxicity through inhibition of mitochondrial DNA polymerase-γ typically cause hepatitis in association with lactic acidosis. This is a feature of some nucleoside reverse transcriptase inhibitors, particularly didanosine and stavudine. Non-alcoholic fatty liver disease also occurs in HIV-positive individuals. Although still associated with traditional risk factors such as raised triglycerides and clinical features such as an increased waist circumference, exposure to nucleoside reverse transcriptase inhibitors may also contribute. In addition, nodular regenerative hyperplasia leading to portal hypertension (non-cirrhotic portal hypertension) has been associated with long-term didanosine use.

## Management of end-stage liver disease

Patients with end-stage chronic liver disease of whatever cause are potential candidates for liver transplantation, usually after their first episode of decompensation. Success rates are related to the cause of the liver disease and the presence of other co-morbidities. The risk of toxicity related to immunosuppressive agents is now better understood and can be avoided by attention to drug interactions and appropriate dose adjustments.

## Conclusions

Liver disease is an important and common co-morbidity in HIV infection, most commonly caused by viral hepatitis. If not already infected, HIV-positive patients should be immunized against hepatitis A and B as soon as possible. There is an epidemic of acute hepatitis C infection among some populations of HIV-positive MSM. They should be screened at least annually for hepatitis C. cART can also contribute to liver damage and patients should be monitored for hepatotoxicity, particularly when starting a new regimen.

## Further reading

British HIV Association. Guidelines on HIV and Co-infection with hepatitis B and C (2010). (www.bhiva.org/documents/Guidelines/HepBC/2010/hiv_781.pdf).

# CHAPTER 12

# Neurological Manifestations

*H. Manji[1] and R. F. Miller[2]*

[1]National Hospital for Neurology, Queen Square, London, UK
[2]University College London, London, UK

---

> **OVERVIEW**
>
> - Primary HIV infection may present with a variety of neurological syndromes including an aseptic meningitis
> - In cART naive patients, the CD4 count still remains a useful guide to aetiology
> - Since the introduction of combination antiretroviral therapy (cART), the incidence of the classical neurological complications of HIV (e.g. cryptococcal meningitis, cerebral toxoplasmosis, progressive multifocal leucoencephalopathy) have decreased
> - Although HIV-associated dementia has declined, there is concern that HIV-associated neurocognitive disorders are increasing despite effective suppression of HIV infection. The aetiology is not well understood and is likely to be multifactorial. Early initiation of cART may be protective.

## Introduction

In patients infected with HIV, all areas of the neuraxis are vulnerable – to HIV itself, opportunistic infections (OIs) and tumours as well some antiretroviral drugs (Box 12.1).

Since the introduction of combination antiretroviral therapy (cART), the incidence of previously encountered OIs and tumours has declined significantly. Although the incidence of severe HIV dementia has decreased, the prevalence of milder forms of neurocognitive impairment has increased. This occurs in a subgroup of patients despite low or negligible viral load in the blood. Patients on cART now present with problems due to drug side effects (e.g. efavirenz causing headaches, drowsiness, agitation, insomnia and cognitive dysfunction), neurological immune reconstitution syndromes and the so-called compartmentalization syndrome with negligible plasma HIV viral loads but high cerebrospinal fluid (CSF) viral loads. Assessment of the impact of HIV and cART on the brain is further complicated by non-HIV-related co-pathology associated with ageing (such as cerebrovascular disease), mental health and alcohol problems associated with persons living with a long-term chronic disease, use of pain control due to complications of HIV disease (e.g. peripheral neuropathy), use of illicit drugs in a subgroup of patients and co-infection with e.g. Hepatitis C.

---

*ABC of HIV and AIDS*, Sixth Edition. Edited by Michael W. Adler,
Simon G. Edwards, Robert F. Miller, Gulshan Sethi and Ian G. Williams.
© 2012 Blackwell Publishing Ltd. Published 2012 by Blackwell Publishing Ltd.

---

> Box 12.1 **Neurological complications in HIV infection**
>
> **Opportunistic infections**
> - *Toxoplasma gondii* – abscesses and encephalitis
> - *Cryptococcus neoformans* – meningitis
> - JC virus – progressive multifocal leucoencephalopathy (PML)
> - CMV – retinitis, encephalitis, cauda equina syndrome, vasculitic neuropathy
> - *Mycobacterium tuberculosis* – meningitis, abscesses
>
> **Tumours**
> - Primary CNS lymphoma (PCNSL)
> - Metastatic systemic lymphoma
>
> **HIV-related disorders**
> - HIV associated neurocognitive disorders (HAND)
> - Vacuolar myelopathy
> - Peripheral neuropathy (distal sensory peripheral neuropathy)
> - Polymyositis
>
> **Drug-induced complications**
> - Neuropathy (didanosine, stavudine, isoniazid)
> - Myalgia, myopathy (NRTIs)
>
> **Immune reconstitution syndromes**
> - *Cryptococcus neoformans*
> - Progressive multifocal leukoencephalopathy (PML)
> - *M. tuberculosis*
> - HIV

Some antiretrovirals may increase vascular risk factors. It is not yet clear whether HIV-infected patients will be more prone to the neurodegenerative disorders associated with ageing such as Alzheimer's and Parkinson's diseases and also primary brain tumours.

## Primary HIV seroconversion illness

At seroconversion, a glandular fever-like illness occurs in 70% of cases. In 10%, this maybe associated with neurological signs and symptoms (Box 12.2). The aseptic meningitis which presents with headache, meningism and seizures is usually self-limiting. An acute demyelinating polyradiculoneuropathy (Guillain–Barré syndrome) is identical to that found in non-infected individuals both clinically and in the response to treatment with intravenous immunoglobulin and or plasma exchange. The only clue maybe a pleocytosis of >20 cells/μL, which would be unusual in non HIV cases.

---

Box 12.2 **Neurological syndromes at seroconversion**

- Aseptic meningitis
- Meningoencephalitis
- Acute disseminated encephalomyelitis (ADEM)
- Transverse myelitis
- Cauda equina syndrome
- Acute demyelinating polyradiculoneuropathy (Guillain–Barré syndrome)
- Brachial neuritis
- Mononeuritis multiplex (vasculitis)
- Acute polymyositis

---

A high index of suspicion is required in all such presentations and testing for HIV infection should always be offered (see Chapters 3 and 4 for most appropriate tests to perform during primary HIV seroconversion illness).

## Asymptomatic HIV disease

During the asymptomatic phase of the illness, headache and cranial nerve palsies (especially the VIIth nerve) may be the only manifestation of a chronic low-grade meningitis. CSF examination during this phase may however show abnormalities with a pleocytosis, an elevated protein level and oligoclonal bands making it necessary to investigate infections such as syphilis with specific tests such as the venereal disease research laboratory (VDRL) test and the *Treponema pallidum* haemagglutination (TPHA) test.

Large cohort studies have conclusively demonstrated no evidence of HIV dementia developing during this asymptomatic, immunocompetent phase.

## Advanced HIV disease

### General principles

The CD4 count is a useful guide to the aetiology of a neurological presentation in patients not on cART – toxoplasmosis and cryptococcal meningitis occur at CD4 counts <200 cells/μL whereas complications due to cytomegalovirus (CMV) mainly occur at CD4 counts <50 cells/μL.

Since HIV itself results in cytochemical CSF changes, the diagnosis of encephalitis and meningitis requires specific tests to identify the cause, e.g. cryptococcal latex agglutination (CrAg), JCV or herpesviruses by polymerase chain reaction (PCR).

The intrathecal inflammatory response is impaired – hence patients with meningitis may not present with typical signs of meningism such as neck stiffness, photophobia and Kernig's sign. The threshold for performing computed tomography/magnetic resonance imaging (CT/MRI) followed by lumbar puncture is necessarily low.

The measurement of serum antibodies to diagnose, for example toxoplasmosis, is unhelpful since the rise in immunoglobulin (Ig)M levels may not occur.

Infection with more than one organism may occur, for example *Cryptococcus neoformans* and *Mycobacterium tuberculosis*, and this needs to be considered in cases where there is lack of therapeutic response or deterioration after initial improvement. Opportunistic infections in the brain are rare in patients on successful cART.

The two main presentations of opportunistic disease of the brain in individuals with advanced HIV infection are discussed below.

## Meningitis (Box 12.3)

The commonest cause of meningitis in HIV-infected patients is *Cryptococcus neoformans*. Patients present with general malaise, headache, confusion or seizures that have an acute or insidious onset over days or weeks. The classical signs of meningism are frequently absent. Brain imaging is usually normal but may reveal hydrocephalus, or cryptococcomas (dilated Virchow-Robin spaces which are filled with the fungal organism). The CSF cell count, protein and glucose maybe normal. The diagnosis is confirmed by the detection of cryptococcal antigen in CSF in >95% of cases. India ink staining is positive in 75% and culture is positive in ≤85%.

---

Box 12.3 **Meningitis in HIV infection**

**Fungal**
- *Cryptococcus neoformans*

**Bacterial**
- *Streptococcus pneumoniae*
- *Mycobacterium tuberculosis*

**Viral**
- *Herpes simplex*
- *Varicella zoster*

---

At lumbar puncture, it is essential to perform manometry as the opening pressure is frequently raised. Intracranial hypertension in the absence of mass lesions or hydrocephalus is a significant cause of mortality and visual failure. This is due to blockage of CSF resorption across the ventricular arachnoid villi by *Cryptococcus*. Several features associated with a poor outcome have been identified (Box 12.4).

---

Box 12.4 **Poor prognostic features in HIV-associated Cryptococcal meningitis**

- Altered mental status
  - obtundation
  - coma
- CSF white cell count <20 lymphocytes/μL
- CSF opening pressure >25 cm CSF
- CSF CrAg >1:1000
- Positive India ink or mucicarmine staining
- Hyponatraemia
- Culture of extrameningeal *Cryptococcus* e.g. in blood or from skin
- Relapse episode

---

The mainstay of treatment consists of a 2-week induction period with liposomal amphotericin B, usually combined with flucytosine followed by 6 weeks of fluconazole. Management of raised intracranial pressure is by repeated lumbar puncture; occasionally insertion of an external ventricular or lumbar drain is necessary. There are no data to support use of acetazolamide or steroids.

## Presentation with focal neurology

Patients may present with focal neurological symptoms and signs and or seizures as a result of infections (toxoplasmosis, JC virus, *M. tuberculosis*, CMV, herpes simplex and varicella zoster), tumours (primary CNS lymphoma (PCNSL)) and cerebrovascular disease, which also includes meningitis-associated vasculitis (Figure 12.1).

The commonest causes of mass lesions (space-occupying lesions with cerebral oedema) on imaging are toxoplasmosis, PCNSL and *M. tuberculosis*

Progressive multifocal leucoencephalopthy (PML) due to JC virus encephalitis due to the herpesviruses and stroke usually cause focal imaging abnormalities without associated mass effect.

## Toxoplasmosis

In HIV infection, toxoplasmosis is usually a reactivation of latent infection in individuals who have previously been exposed to the organism. The clinical presentation is usually with headache with rapidly evolving focal neurological deficits over 1–2 weeks – hemiparesis, dysphasia, visual field deficits, movement disorders (chorea/athetosis, parkinsonism) and seizures. A diffuse encephalitis has also been described. Rarely, toxoplasmosis may affect the spinal cord and present with a myelopathy or a cauda equina syndrome.

Blood serology for *Toxoplasma gondii* is only helpful if negative, since this makes the diagnosis less likely. Patients should have their toxoplasmosis serology documented at the first diagnosis of HIV infection. Prior to the availability of cART, the risk of developing toxoplasma encephalitis in IgG seropositive patients was between 12% and 30%. These patients should be offered primary prophylaxis with co-trimoxazole at CD4 counts <200 cells/μL. This can be stopped when patients on cART have a CD4 count >200 cells/μL for 6 months.

CT/MRI shows multiple enhancing lesions with mass effect in the region of the basal ganglia and at the grey–white interface (Figure 12.2). A response to treatment is usually seen in 80% by day 14. Providing there is continued improvement, it is reasonable to repeat imaging 4–6 weeks after starting treatment. In patients with significant mass effect on scans and symptoms of raised intracranial pressure such as altered conscious level, severe headache, vomiting, neck stiffness and papilloedema, additional

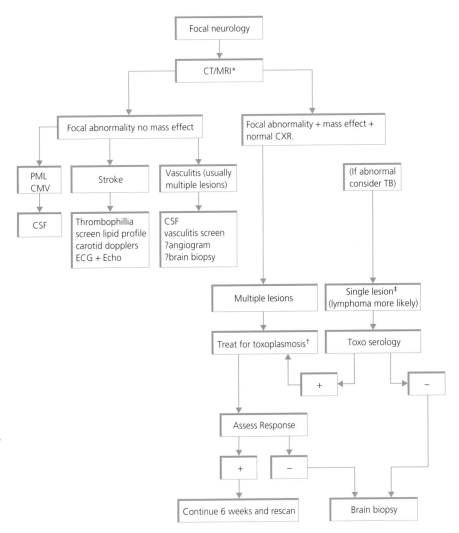

**Figure 12.1** Flow chart showing investigation pathways for patients with mass lesions on magnetic resonance imaging (MRI). *MRI preferred – increased sensitivity especially for posterior fossa lesions. †Treat with dexamethasone if symptoms and signs of ↑ ICP. ‡Thallium SPECT scans may help differentiate between lymphoma and abscess with increased uptake in the lymphoma. CMV, cytomegalovirus; PML, progressive multifocal leucoencephalopthy; CSF, cerebrospinal fluid.

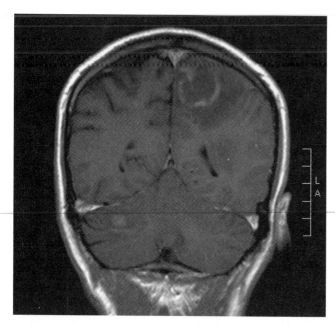

**Figure 12.2** Toxoplasmosis. Lesion at grey/white interface in the parietal lobe and in the cerebellum.

treatment with dexamethasone is indicated. This will, however, confound the assessment of response to treatment since any observed clinical or radiological improvement may be due to the steroids. Clinical deterioration should prompt consideration of a brain biopsy.

### Primary CNS lymphoma

PCNSL is the second most common cause of mass lesions in HIV-infected adults (Figure 12.3). The diagnosis of PCNSL is made by brain biopsy (see Chapter 7).

### Progressive multifocal leucoencephalopthy

PML results from a reactivation of the JC virus in immunosuppressed individuals. Over 80% of the population will have been exposed to the virus in childhood and will be seropositive in blood samples.

The presentation is with slowly evolving focal neurological deficits such as hemiparesis, visual field defects, language problems and incoordination due to cerebellar involvement. Occasional patients develop dementia with focal neurological signs. Symptoms and signs of raised intracranial pressure are absent although headache may be a feature.

Blood serological testing is unhelpful. Cranial MRI shows non-enhancing areas of low attenuation in the white matter on $T_1$-weighted images and hyperintense lesions on $T_2$-weighted images with typical areas of scalloping at the grey/white interface (Figure 12.4). There is usually no associated oedema. The diagnosis is confirmed by isolating JC virus DNA by PCR in the CSF in $\leq 75\%$ of cases. In patients on cART, the sensitivity is reduced to 30%. Repeat CSF analysis maybe necessary before resorting to brain biopsy.

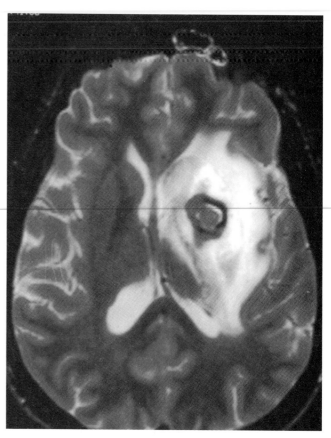

**Figure 12.3** Primary central nervous system lymphoma. Single lesion adjacent to ventricle with surrounding oedema and 'mass effect'.

The treatment of PML pivots around improving immune function with cART. Other treatment strategies directed against JC virus infection have not been shown to confer additional benefit.

### CMV encephalitis

Over 90% of HIV-infected individuals have serological evidence of previous CMV infection. The neurological complications of CMV are thought to be due to reactivation of the virus at low CD4 counts, typically $<50$ cells/$\mu$L. Before the advent of cART, evidence of CMV infection was often found in the brains of patients dying of AIDS. CMV encephalitis should be considered in patients presenting with a rapidly evolving encephalitis involving the brain stem with cranial nerve palsies and seizures. CMV DNA may be isolated from the CSF using PCR. The treatment of choice is ganciclovir, with or without foscarnet.

### HIV-associated neurocognitive disorder (HAND)

Prior to the availability of cART, severe progressive neurocognitive impairment was associated with advanced HIV infection. Since the introduction of cART, the incidence has significantly declined. However, the prevalence of less severe neurocognitive problems has increased, although the aetiology is less well understood.

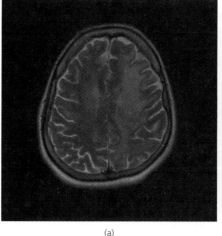 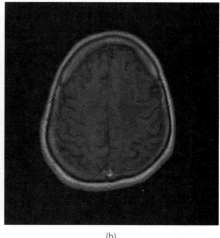

(a)  (b)

**Figure 12.4** Progressive multifocal leucoencephalopthy. (a) $T_2$-weighed image (b) $T_1$-weighted image.

HAND represents a group of syndromes of varying severity affecting cognition, behaviour and motor function. The spectrum ranges from mild asymptomatic neuropsychological impairment (ANI), which is defined by cognitive impairment at least one SD below the mean in two or more cognitive domains without difficulties in activities of daily living, to HIV-associated mild neurocognitive disorder (MND), which is defined as cognitive impairment at least one SD below the mean in two or more cognitive domains accompanied by mild difficulties in activities of daily living. The most severe form is known as HIV-associated dementia (HAD), which was previously known as AIDS dementia complex (ADC). This is defined as marked cognitive impairment at least two SD below the mean in two or more cognitive domains causing moderate-to-severe difficulties in activities of daily living. Clinical features and differential diagnosis of patients presenting with cognitive symptoms are shown in Boxes 12.5 and 12.6.

---

Box 12.5 **Symptoms of HIV-associated mild neurocognitive disorder (MND) and HIV-associated dementia (HAD)**

Neuropsychological assessment is necessary

**HIV-associated mild neurocognitive disorder (MND)**

Patients may complain of:

- difficulty with complex tasks
- mild memory problems
- distractibility/confusion
- need to make lists
- problems with drug adherence

Patient displays at least two of the following symptoms for >1 month:

- impaired attention/concentration
- mental slowing
- slowed movements
- impaired concentration
- personality change, irritability or emotional lability

---

**HIV-associated dementia (HAD)**

Patients or carers may complain of:

- memory problems
- distractibility, poor attention and concentration
- emotional lability
- psychomotor slowing
- poor balance, clumsiness
- social withdrawal
- difficulty with information processing
- language problems
- visuospatial problems
- difficulty with complex motor tasks (apraxias)
- late stages
  - psychotic symptoms
  - severe memory loss
  - seizures
  - myoclonus

Patient displays at least two of the following cognitive symptoms for >1 month:

- impaired attention/concentration
- slowing in processing information
- difficulty with abstraction/reasoning
- difficulty with visuo-spatial skills
- impaired memory and learning
- impaired language function

and at least one of the following:

- acquired abnormality in motor function by clinical testing (e.g. myelopathy) or neuropsychological testing
- decline in motivation,, emotional control or social behaviour

Risk factors for HAND include older age, female gender, current or previous low CD4 count (<100 cells/μL), high plasma HIV viral load, co-morbid conditions (e.g. anaemia), co-infection with hepatitis C and history of injection drug use. The diagnosis is one of exclusion of other infective, neoplastic, metabolic and

**Table 12.1** Central nervous system penetration effectiveness (CPE) score.

| Drug class | CPE score | | | |
|---|---|---|---|---|
| | 4 | 3 | 2 | 1 |
| NRTI | Zidovudine | Abacavir<br>Emtricitabine | Didanosine<br>Lamivudine<br>Stavudine | Tenofovir<br>Zalcitabine |
| NNRTI | Nevirapine | Delavirdine<br>Efavirenz | Etravirine | |
| PI | B/Indinavir | B/Darunavir<br>B/Fosamprenavir<br>B/Lopinavir<br>Indinavir | Atazanavir<br>B/Atazanavir<br>Fosamprenavir | Nelfinavir<br>Ritonavir<br>Saquinavir<br>B/Saquinavir<br>B/Tipranavir |
| Entry/fusion inhibitors | | Maraviroc | | Enfuvirtide |
| Integrase inhibitors | | Raltegravir | | |

B, boosted (with ritonavir).

iatrogenic aetiologies by brain imaging and CSF examination. Although there is a correlation between CSF HIV RNA viral load and severity of dementia, there is too much overlap for use as a diagnostic test. Cranial MRI shows variable cortical atrophy and diffuse or patchy white matter signal abnormalities on $T_2$-weighted images (Figure 12.5). The nature and extent of MRI changes do not correlate with the clinical severity. A neuropsychological assessment may be useful for objective monitoring of response to treatment.

With the introduction of cART, the incidence of HAND has declined significantly. There is evidence that systemic viral suppression by cART may prevent, halt progression and indeed improve some of the cognitive abnormalities as well as MRI changes. There is concern that a subgroup of patients continues to deteriorate cognitively as a result of ongoing smouldering, low-grade inflammation and neuronal destruction despite adequate systemic viral suppression. The pattern of dementia seems to be a combination of a cortical and subcortical dysfunction.

CSF drug concentrations of antiretrovirals are much lower than plasma concentrations. It is not clear how CSF concentrations reflect parenchymal levels. Certain combinations seem more effective at suppression of CSF HIV levels. A relatively arbitrary CNS penetration score has been developed which may serve as a useful guide when faced with a patient with progressive dementia despite systemic viral suppression (Table 12.1).

## Peripheral nerve disorders in HIV infection

### Distal sensory peripheral neuropathy (Box 12.7)

Prior to the introduction of cART, up to 40% of patients developed distal sensory peripheral neuropathy (DSPN). A further 40% had subclinical involvement as shown on nerve biopsy (Boxes 12.7 and 12.8). Treatment is symptomatic with anticonvulsants (gabapentin, pregabalin, lamotrigine, carbamazepine), antidepressants (amitriptyline) and opiates (oxycodone). In patients with a progressive neuropathy apart from considering vasculitis, there is evidence for screening and treating aspects of the metabolic syndrome (hyperglycaemia, hypertriglyceridaemia and hypercholesterolaemia).

### Antiretroviral toxic neuropathy

This neuropathy, primarily due to the nucleoside analogue drugs didanosine and stavudine, is dose dependent and presents with similar symptoms and signs to DSPN. It is usually a more painful neuropathy than DSPN.

Approximately 60% of patients improve on stopping the drug but others are left with neuropathic symptoms, most likely due to the unmasking of an underlying DSPN especially if the CD4 count

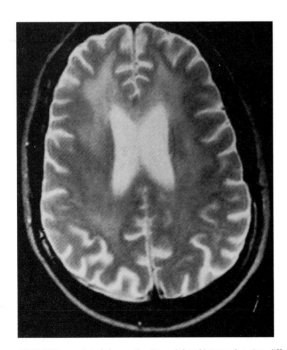

**Figure 12.5** HIV-associated dementia. $T_2$-weighted image showing diffuse and multiple areas of white matter demyelination with no mass effect.

was <200 cells/mm$^3$ for any length of time prior to starting drug treatment.

Investigation of HIV neuropathy is shown in Box 12.9.

---

**Box 12.7 Peripheral nerve disorders in HIV infection**

**HIV related**

- Distal sensory peripheral neuropathy (DSPN)
- Demyelinating neuropathy

    - acute – Guillain–Barré syndrome
    - chronic – Chronic inflammatory demyelinating polyneuropathy (CIDP)

- Vasculitic neuropathy – mononeuritis multiplex
- Diffuse infiltrative lymphocytosis syndrome (DILS)
- Motor neuron disease like syndrome

**CMV related**

- Vasculitic neuropathy - mononeuritis multiplex
- Lumbosacral polyradiculopathy

**Drug induced**

- didanosine, stavudine
- isoniazid
- thalidomide
- dapsone
- metronidazole

---

**Box 12.8 Symptoms and signs of DSPN**

- Numb, burning feet
- Sharp stabbing pains
- Contact hypersensitivity
- Little or no weakness
- Impaired pain and temperature sensation
- Normal, depressed or absent ankle reflexes

---

**Box 12.9 Work up of HIV neuropathy**

- Consider neurotoxic drugs, including excess vitamin B$_6$
- Consider excess alcohol and poor diet
- Blood tests: Vitamin B$_{12}$, fasting glucose, HbA$_1$C and oral glucose tolerance test, VDRL. In patients >60 years old – immunoglobulins, serum protein electrophoresis, urine for Bence–Jones protein (for myeloma and amyloid), anti-neuronal antibodies (for paraneoplastic neuropathy)
- Nerve conduction tests – indicated if weakness > toe extension (extensor hallucis longus), significant large fibre involvement (joint position and vibration), asymmetric presentation or severe pain
- Nerve biopsy – usually sural nerve looking for vasculitis, DILS, CIDP, malignant infiltration

---

## Neurological IRIS syndromes

Immune reconstitution inflammatory syndrome (IRIS) following initiation of cART is increasingly recognized. The consequences of IRIS occurring in the brain can be devastating. CNS IRIS occurs with opportunistic infections such as cryptococcal (Figure 12.6), PML (Figure 12.7) and TB meningitis, although it may also occur in a wide variety of HIV-related CNS disease (Figure 12.7) (Box 12.10).

The management of neurological IRIS is controversial. The standard strategy is to treat the underlying infection (if present) and treat the associated mass effect and oedema with steroids such as dexamethasone.

Despite the success of cART, neurological disorders in patients with good CD4 counts and undetectable viral loads are increasingly encountered. Examples include:

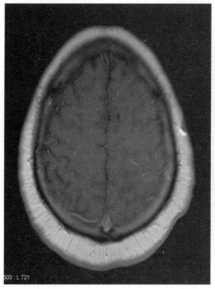
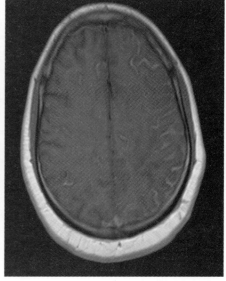

**Figure 12.6** Cryptococccal immune reconstitution inflammatory syndrome with diffuse meningeal enhancement: MR appearances (a) before starting cART and (b) after starting cART.

(a)　　　　　　　　　　　　　(b)

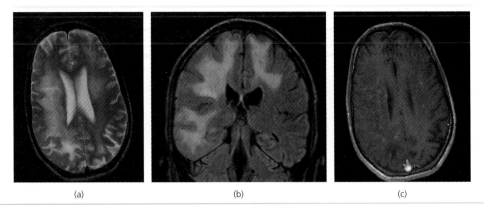

**Figure 12.7** Progressive multifocal leucoencephalopthy IRIS showing diffuse enhancement.

Box 12.10 **Neurological IRIS**

**OI associated**

- PML
- *M. tuberculosisis* (meningitis, tuberculoma)
- *C. neoformans* (meningitis, intracranial cryptococcomas)
- Herpesvirus (VZV, CMV, HSV, EBV) (encephalitis, cerebral vasculitis, retinitis, stroke, optic neuritis)
- Toxoplasmosis (encephalitis)
  - 'unmasked IRIS' – reactivation of latent infection due to immune restoration.
  - 'paradoxical IRIS' – known infection e.g. PML. Deterioration after initiation of cART

**HIV associated**

- Subacute generalized encephalopathy (altered mental status, seizures, coma). MRI: multifocal diffuse high signal on $T_2$ and flair images. Histopathology: massive CNS CD8 infiltration.
- Acute inflammatory demyelinating encephalitis (MS like)
- Vasculitis
- Chronic HIV associated CNS IRIS causing HAND
- Guillain–Barré syndrome

- An HIV compartmentalization syndrome where the CSF HIV viral load is much higher than plasma viral load. Patients may present acutely or subacutely with increasing confusion, ataxia and cognitive decline (Figure 12.8).
- Acute HIV IRIS, which presents with an encephalitis-like syndrome.
- Chronic HIV IRIS syndrome, which presents insidiously with headache, seizures and focal neurological deficits and which may or may not be associated with a CNS vasculitis.

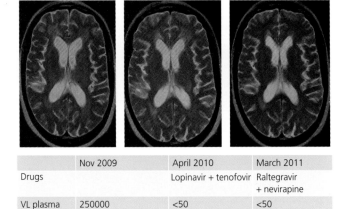

|  | Nov 2009 | April 2010 | March 2011 |
|---|---|---|---|
| Drugs |  | Lopinavir + tenofovir | Raltegravir + nevirapine |
| VL plasma | 250000 | <50 | <50 |
| VL CSF |  | 1400 | <50 |

**Figure 12.8** HIV compartmentalization syndrome.

## Further reading

Garvey L, Winston A, Walsh J, *et al*; UK Collaborative HIV Cohort (CHIC) study. Antiretroviral therapy CNS penetration and HIV-1-associated CNS disease. *Neurology* 2011;76:693–700.

Gonzalez-Duarte A, Cikurel K, Simpson DM. Managing HIV peripheral neuropathy. *Curr HIV/AIDS Rep* 2007;4:114–118.

Manji H, Miller R. The neurology of HIV infection. *J Neurol Neurosurg Psychiatry* 2004;75(Suppl 1):i29–35.

Schouten J, Cinque P, Gisslen M *et al*. HIV-1 infection and cognitive impairment in the cART era: A Review. *AIDS* 2011, 25:561–575.

Valcour V, Paul R, Chiao S, Wendelken LA, Miller B. Screening for cognitive impairment in human immunodeficiency virus. *Clin Infect Dis* 2011;53: 836–842.

Weissert R. Progressive multifocal leukoencephalopathy *J Neuroimmunol* 2011;231:73–77.

# CHAPTER 13

# The Eye and HIV

*C. Younan[1], W. Lynn[2] and S. Lightman[3]*

[1]Westmead and Sydney Eye Hospitals, Sydney, Australia
[2]Ealing Hospital, London, UK
[3]Moorfields Eye Hospital, London, UK

## OVERVIEW

- For patients with HIV infection, the risk and pattern of eye involvement alter with the level of immune function, and in particular with the CD4 count
- In HIV-infected individuals cotton wool spots, retinal microaneurysms and retinal haemorrhages can occur in the absence of opportunistic infection or alternative pathology
- Sexually transmitted infections are a common cause of presentation to an ophthalmologist

## Introduction

Patients with HIV infection are at increased risk of infectious or malignant pathologies that can involve multiple organs, including the eye. The risk and pattern of eye involvement alters with the level of immune function, and in particular with the CD4 count. Patients with a CD4 count greater than 500 cells/µL are often asymptomatic, but may have inflammatory eye conditions such as allergic conjunctivitis. When the CD4 count is between 200 and 500 cells/µL, ocular bacterial infections become more prominent. At levels below 200 cells/µL there is a significant risk of developing opportunistic infections or malignancy, and this is of particular concern when the count is below 75 cells/µL.

There are a number of common causes of a patient infected with HIV presenting with a red eye or with vision loss, and these are summarized in Tables 13.1 and 13.2 respectively. The appearance of some ocular infections may be sufficiently characteristic to allow an immediate clinical diagnosis to be made. Thus dilated fundoscopic evaluation can be invaluable in the investigation of the febrile immunocompromised patient.

## Non-infectious HIV retinopathy

There are several retinal findings within the eye that may be present at any stage of untreated HIV infection. These include cotton wool spots (Figure 13.1), retinal microaneurysms and retinal haemorrhages, and do not necessarily reflect an opportunistic

*ABC of HIV and AIDS*, Sixth Edition. Edited by Michael W. Adler,
Simon G. Edwards, Robert F. Miller, Gulshan Sethi and Ian G. Williams.
© 2012 Blackwell Publishing Ltd. Published 2012 by Blackwell Publishing Ltd.

**Table 13.1** Common causes of a red eye.

| Cause | Typical symptoms or signs | Typically painful | Typically associated with vision loss |
|---|---|---|---|
| Blepharitis | Itchy, burning eyes | No | No |
| Conjunctivitis | Chemosis and discharge | No | No |
| Keratitis | Loss of corneal clarity | Yes | Yes |
| Episcleritis | Chemosis | Yes | No |
| Anterior scleritis | Chemosis | Markedly | No |
| Anterior uveitis | Floaters | Minimally | Varies with degree of inflammation |

**Table 13.2** Common causes of vision loss.

| Cause | Typical symptoms or signs | Typically associated with pain |
|---|---|---|
| Keratitis | Loss of corneal clarity | Yes |
| Posterior scleritis | Pain with eye movement | Yes |
| Uveitis – anterior | Red eye | No |
| Uveitis – intermediate | Floaters | No |
| Uveitis – posterior | Acute onset of vision loss | No |
| Retinitis | Acute onset of vision loss | No |
| Optic neuropathy | Colour vision affected | No |

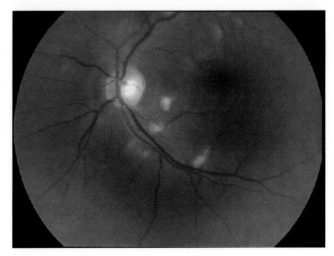

**Figure 13.1** Cotton wool spots as seen in HIV retinopathy.

infection or alternative pathology. These changes are a direct result of HIV infection itself and are not seen when patients are successfully treated with combination antiretroviral therapy (cART).

## Ocular infection associated with HIV

### Cytomegalovirus

Cytomegalovirus (CMV) retinitis (Figure 13.2) is by far the most common ocular opportunistic infection in patients with HIV infection. The annual risk of retinitis is reported as being as high as 20% when the CD4 count drops below 50 cells/μL. With current cART both newly diagnosed CMV retinitis and disease relapses have been markedly reduced. The ability for recent cART to restore immune function has been pivotal to this change.

If the CMV retinitis is located at or close to the macula or optic nerve the risk of vision loss is high. Intraocular injections of either ganciclovir or foscarnet may be used. A ganciclovir implant placed

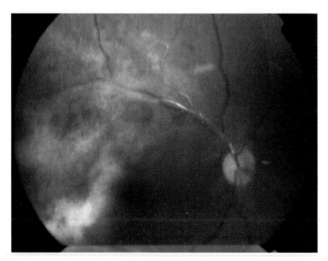

**Figure 13.2** Cytomegalovirus retinitis.

within the patient's affected eye (Figure 13.3) releases drug over a 6-month period and reduces the need for repeated intraocular injections. Intraocular therapy will only protect the affected eye and systemic anti-CMV therapy is still required to prevent disease in the uninvolved eye and treat or prevent CMV disease in other parts of the body. Oral valganciclovir is the preferred systemic anti-CMV therapy, but intravenous ganciclovir or foscarnet can be considered if there are potential issues with adherence, absorption or specific contraindications to oral therapy. Intravenous cidofovir is an alternative, but its use is limited by nephrotoxicity and may also be complicated by an inflammatory reaction with the CMV infected eye. Dosing regimens are summarized in Table 13.3.

Patients on cART are usually able to discontinue maintenance anti-CMV therapy once there is confirmation of inactive retinal disease and good HIV virological control with a sustained immunological improvement (e.g. CD4 count >100 cells/μL for at least 3 months). While the risk of relapse of CMV retinitis relates to the level of immune function, the risk of retinal detachment does not, and can occur months after the retinal disease has been controlled. The greater the area of retinitis, the greater the risk of retinal detachment. Immune recovery uveitis may also be seen. This is a cART-dependent response and can itself reduce vision.

### Herpes simplex virus

This virus may affect either the anterior or posterior segment of the eye. Herpes simplex virus (HSV) keratitis (Figure 13.4) may permanently affect vision if the centre of the cornea is involved and

**Table 13.3** Drug therapy for cytomegalovirus retinitis.

| Drug | Induction dose | Maintenance dose | Intravitreal dose |
|------|---------------|------------------|-------------------|
| Ganciclovir | 6 mg/kg bd iv | 5–6 mg/kg daily iv | 2 mg in 0.1 mL |
| Valganciclovir | 900 mg bd po | 900 mg daily po | N/A |
| Foscarnet | 90 mg/kg bd iv | 90 mg/kg daily iv | 2.4 mg in 0.1 mL |

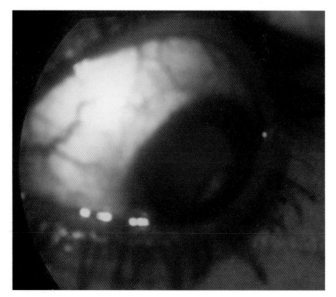

**Figure 13.3** Ganciclovir implant inside eye.

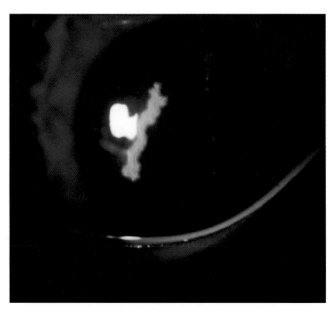

**Figure 13.4** Herpes simplex keratitis stained with fluorescein.

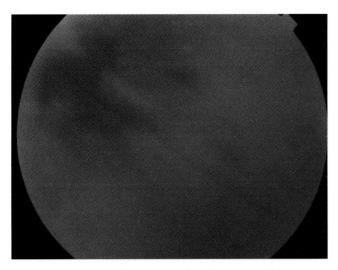

**Figure 13.5** Acute retinal necrosis – note that the retina a is white.

is usually treated with topical aciclovir ointment. HSV involving the retina causes acute retinal necrosis (Figure 13.5) and can result in rapid vision loss if treatment is not initiated quickly. The virus can be confirmed by polymerase chain reaction analysis of a vitreous sample, at which time the patient can be given an intravitreal foscarnet injection. Treatment is continued with intravenous aciclovir for at least 7 days followed by oral aciclovir for 6 weeks, but oral valaciclovir may be able to replace the intravenous treatment. Unlike CMV retinitis, HSV retinitis can occur at higher CD4 counts, and is also seen in patients who are immunocompetent.

## Varicella zoster virus

This virus can cause multiple ophthalmic disorders. With herpes zoster ophthalmicus, the eyelids and conjunctiva may become

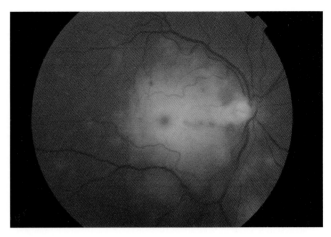

**Figure 13.7** Varicella zoster virus retinitis.

red and swollen (Figure 13.6). Cerebral vasculitis may cause cranial nerve palsies and disorders of extraocular movement. Ocular involvement may be as a keratitis, uveitis or necrotizing retinitis. Varicella zoster virus (VZV) can cause acute retinal necrosis similar to that seen with HSV infection and is treated similarly. However, in patients with very low CD4 counts (usually less than 10 cells/μL), an aggressive, rapidly progressive retinitis (previously known as progressive outer retinal necrosis or PORN) may occur (Figure 13.7). Multiple discrete retinal lesions rapidly coalesce and cause very rapid total retinal destruction with little associated ocular inflammation. Treatment involves intravitreal foscarnet at the time of vitreous sampling, followed by intravenous high-dose aciclovir, foscarnet or ganciclovir. The incidence of retinal detachment is high and the prognosis for vision is very poor.

## Toxoplasmosis

Retinitis due to *Toxoplasma gondii* may occur as a primary infection or most commonly as reactivation of previously acquired ocular infection (Figure 13.8). It is more likely to occur with CD4 counts less than 150 cells/μL. Anterior uveitis and vitritis are often, but

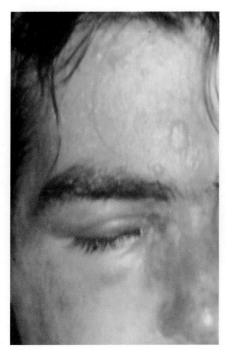

**Figure 13.6** Herpes zoster ophthalmicus.

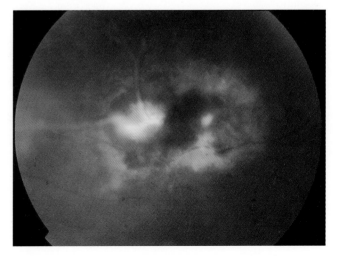

**Figure 13.8** Recurrent retinal toxoplasmosis infection at edge of scar.

not necessarily, present. Cerebral imaging is indicated because of the frequency of associated central nervous system disease (29% of patients in one study). Treatment of ocular toxoplasmosis uses the same drug regimens as those employed for cerebral disease, i.e. sulfadiazine plus pyrimethamine. Acute therapy should continue until the retinal lesion is quiescent (and coexisting cerebral disease is under control) and secondary prophylaxis should be continued until the CD4 count is maintained above 200 cells/μL.

## Tuberculosis

Within the eye tuberculosis (TB) can present with uveitis or, less commonly, ocular granulomas. The characteristic appearance of choroidal granulomata in TB (Figure 13.9) may be useful in helping to establish a clinical diagnosis of tuberculosis in the febrile HIV patient. Ocular TB granulomas do not require any specific ocular treatment and will respond to standard systemic antituberculous therapy. Ocular TB uveitis requires topical (for anterior uveitis) or systemic (for intermediate or posterior uveitis) steroid therapy.

## Syphilis

Syphilis may affect any part of the eye and simulate many other disease processes. The periorbital tissues may be inflamed secondary to a chancre from primary infection after direct genital contact. With later stages of infection ocular involvement may be as an anterior uveitis (most common) or posterior uveitis. Marked vitritis is characteristic of co-infection with syphilis and HIV. Patients with ocular syphilis and HIV infection may already be in the tertiary phase of syphilitic infection and need to be investigated and treated as such. With tertiary syphilis, miotic (Argyll Robertson) pupils may be seen, where there is no pupillary response to light, but constriction is noted with accommodation.

## Gonorrhoea

Typically presentation is acute with a markedly purulent conjunctivitis. Without appropriate and timely treatment this may lead to severe vision loss due to corneal scarring or perforation. Systemic antibiotic treatment is required (such as ceftriaxone 1 g im as a single dose), and saline irrigation followed by topical antibiotics is recommended.

## Chlamydia

Adult inclusion conjunctivitis is the most common presentation of ocular infection with *Chlamydia trachomatis*. The typical presentation is a chronic follicular conjunctivitis (with or without mucopurulent discharge) that is usually self limiting, even in the absence of antibiotic therapy. On systemic review these patients are found to have genital tract infection in 50–90% of cases. Both topical (for example tetracycline ointment) and systemic therapy (such as azithromycin 1 g single dose or doxycycline 100 mg bd for 7 days) are required.

Reactive arthritis affects 1–3% of men following genital infection with *C. trachomatis*. The typical triad is of arthritis, urethritis and conjunctivitis and 75–90% will be positive for HLA-B27. Conjunctivitis is the most common ocular association and typically resolves without treatment in 10 days. Uveitis is less common, but requires topical steroid and mydriatic therapy to limit complications that may affect vision.

## Infective choroiditis

HIV patients with systemic infections may have haematogenous spread to the vascular choroidal layer of the eye, causing an infective choroiditis. Thus dilated fundoscopy should be performed in any HIV-infected patient with systemic infection and any visual symptoms. One to several yellow-white lesions are seen at the posterior pole, and are usually asymptomatic. This has been seen with TB, bacterial sepsis, fungal sepsis (such as *Candida*, Figure 13.10) and *Pneumocystis jirovecii*. Treatment is of the underlying infective process with additional intraocular intervention for bacterial and fungal sepsis when the infection has spread from the vascular choroid and retina into the avascular vitreous.

## Cryptococcus

Patients with cryptococcal meningitis may have optic disc swelling which if chronic can lead to optic atrophy. Less commonly multiple choroidal lesions are present that respond to systemic treatment.

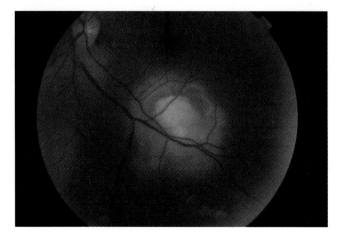

**Figure 13.9** Choroidal tuberculosis.

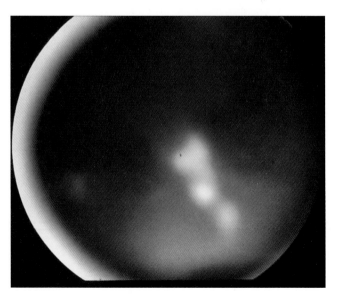

**Figure 13.10** Candida chorioretinitis.

The effect on vision is determined by the degree of optic nerve involvement.

## Malignancy associated with HIV

### Kaposi sarcoma

This sarcoma may involve the eyelids or conjunctiva (Figure 13.11). The lesions usually regress with cART but if not, local excision, cryotherapy, focal irradiation and intralesional injection are alternative treatments.

### Lymphoma

Ocular involvement, when present, is most commonly part of a primary central nervous system (CNS) lymphoma, but the eye may also be involved as part of systemic lymphoma. With primary CNS lymphoma the clinical picture is that of a vitritis, whereas systemic lymphoma usually presents with choroidal involvement or an orbital mass.

### Squamous cell carcinoma of the conjunctiva

This carcinoma is associated with sun exposure and β-HPV infection. They appear as localized, raised, vascular conjunctival lesions

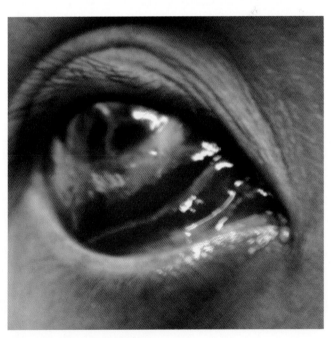

**Figure 13.11** Kaposi sarcoma.

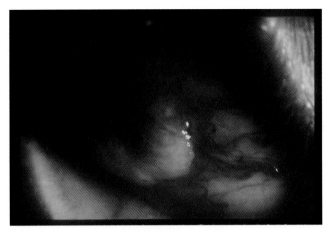

**Figure 13.12** Squamous carcinoma of the conjunctiva.

(Figure 13.12), but can be clinically difficult to distinguish from other conjunctival pathologies. Excisional biopsy is usually recommended.

## Drug-induced ocular disease

Rifabutin is used to treat patients with *Mycobacterium avium intracellulare* (MAI) infection. If rifabutin accumulates within the eye, there is marked intraocular inflammation, which settles with topical steroids and drug dose reduction.

Cidofovir may be used for treatment of CMV retinitis. Its use may also be associated with a marked intraocular inflammatory response, especially in patients on cART.

## Further reading

Holland GN. AIDS and ophthalmology: the first quarter century. *Am J Ophthalmol* 2008;145:397–408.

Jabs DA. Cytomegalovirus retinitis and the acquired immunodeficiency syndrome - bench to bedside: LXVII Edward Jackson Memorial Lecture. *Am J Ophthalmol* 2011;151:198–216.

Nussenblatt RB, Whitcup SM. Acquired immunodeficiency syndrome. In *Uveitis: Fundamentals and Clinical Practice*, 4th edition. Mosby Elsevier, 2010, Chapter 11.

# CHAPTER 14

# The Skin and HIV

*R. Morris-Jones and E. Higgins*

Kings College Hospital, London, UK

---

**OVERVIEW**

- Skin disorders are very common in HIV patients
- Severity of skin disease increases with decreasing CD4 counts
- Cutaneous presentations are often atypical
- Have a low threshold for taking a skin biopsy
- Management of skin diseases is often difficult, but combination antiretroviral therapy usually helps

## Introduction

The skin acts as a window to underlying systemic diseases including HIV and AIDS. The visual nature of cutaneous disorders means they often act as the initial warning sign of impaired immunity. In general, the incidence and severity of skin diseases in HIV patients is inversely proportional to their CD4 count. Common dermatoses such as psoriasis, eczema and acne can present *denovo* in the context of HIV and are often resistant to simple therapies. Managing recalcitrant skin disease in HIV patients over the past decade has been transformed by the advent of cART; however, 70% of patients still suffer from HIV-related skin problems with a high incidence of drug rashes and challenging immune reconstitution syndrome. Physicians should have a low threshold for performing a skin biopsy in HIV patients with skin disease as opportunistic infections (CMV, coccidioidomycosis), rare diseases and atypical presentations of common conditions manifest.

## Seborrhoeic dermatitis

An immunological shift in the host–commensal relationship is thought to trigger an eczematous reaction to the yeast *Malassezia furfur* on the skin. Seborrhoeic dermatitis (SD) affects approximately 1–3% of the general population compared with 50% of HIV-positive patients. Immune dysregulation caused by HIV itself it thought to contribute to the high incidence, particularly in individuals with CD4 counts <100 cells/μL. Classically SD affects the

*ABC of HIV and AIDS*, Sixth Edition. Edited by Michael W. Adler,
Simon G. Edwards, Robert F. Miller, Gulshan Sethi and Ian G. Williams.
© 2012 Blackwell Publishing Ltd. Published 2012 by Blackwell Publishing Ltd.

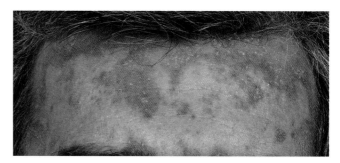

**Figure 14.1** Seborrhoeic dermatitis. Erythema with greasy scale on the forehead.

scalp (Figure 14.1), eyebrows/moustache, nasal creases and anterior chest. The eruption is usually asymptomatic. SD is diagnosed on clinical features; however, large numbers of *Malassezia* yeast can be visualized on microscopy from scrapings. Adherent scalp scale can be lifted by an application of emollient overnight. Twice weekly ketoconazole shampoo to affected skin/scalp can help prevent the scaly eczematous reaction. A combination of hydrocortisone 1% with miconazole nitrate used twice daily is usually effective at relieving the eczema; however, SD is a chronic disease that recurs. Very severe cases of SD in the context of HIV infection can be treated with systemic imidazoles, but complete resolution may only occur following the initiation of cART.

## Kaposi sarcoma

Human herpesvirus type 8 is associated with the pathogenesis of Kaposi sarcoma (KS). In the context of HIV cutaneous KS lesions usually affects the face, oral cavity and perineum. Early lesions may be erythematous-violaceous patches or papules that progress to firm plaques, nodules (Figure 14.2) and eventually ulcers with a purplish-brown discoloration. Lesions can occur at sites of trauma (koebnerize), and secondary lymphoedema may occur. Mucocutaneous KS should be confirmed histologically. Radiological imaging may be required to look for systemic involvement. Cutaneous therapy is aimed at controlling bleeding, functionality, cosmetically disturbing and bulky disease. A variety of measures can be considered such as excision, radiotherapy, pulsed-dye laser and intralesional chemotherapy (vinblastine, vincristine and bleomycin).

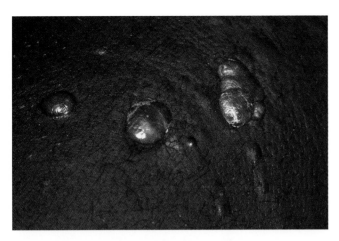

**Figure 14.2** Kaposi sarcoma. Purplish-red firm nodules.

## Pruritic papular eruption/eosinophilic folliculitis

An intensely pruritic follicular eruption of unknown cause that typically manifests when CD4 counts <250 cells/μL. Multiple discrete, erythematous, perifollicular, papules and pustules affect the face and trunk (Figure 14.3). Differential diagnoses include *Staphylococcus*

or *Pityrosporum* folliculitis and acne. Microbiological swabs are negative. Peripheral eosinophilia and raised immunoglobulin E may be seen. Skin biopsy shows characteristic perifollicular mast cells and degranulating eosinophils. cART is an effective treatment when CD4 counts rise >250 cells/μL. UV-B phototherapy can be effective, as are moderately potent topical corticosteroids and permethrin. Systemic indomethacin, minocycline and itraconazole have been used successfully.

## Nodular prurigo

Non-specific pruritus is common in HIV patients, 30% developing nodular prurigo, the cause of which is unknown. Lesions start as small red papules on the trunk and limbs which itch intensely and through scratching develop into chronic nodules (Figure 14.4) that are scarred and hyperpigmented. Nodular prurigo can be very persistent and responds poorly to most treatments. Patients should use a regular emollient to combat dryness and itching. Moderately potent topical steroids applied daily under occlusion may flatten lesions and reduce itching. UVB phototherapy, ciclosporin and amitriptyline may be helpful.

## Drug rashes

The frequency of drug rashes in HIV patients is 10 times higher than in the general population, especially at CD4 counts <200 cells/μL. HIV patients often take multiple medications simultaneously, and HIV itself affects the metabolism of many drugs. The majority of drug rashes occur 7–20 days after commencement of the offending drug, and take the form of toxic erythema, which is usually mild and resolves when the medication is stopped. Emtricitabine (FTC) is one of the most widely prescribed anti-HIV medications. It has been reported to cause skin pigmentation (SP), the incidence of which varies with ethnicity, with a higher rate in African-American patients (8%). Zidovudine is also associated with pigmentation of nails/tongue/skin. Use of abacavir may lead to the development of a hypersensitivity reaction, which usually appears within the first 6 weeks. This usually presents as diffuse erythema

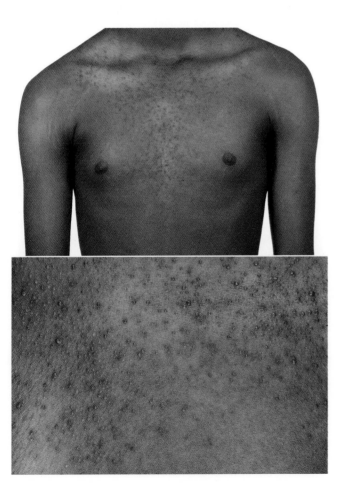

**Figure 14.3** Eosinophilic folliculitis. Papules and pustules around hair follicles on the chest.

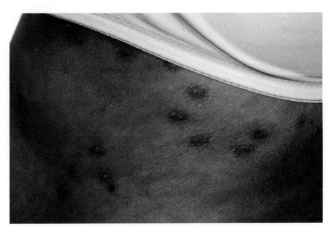

**Figure 14.4** Nodular prurigo. Multiple excoriated hyperpigmented nodules on the trunk.

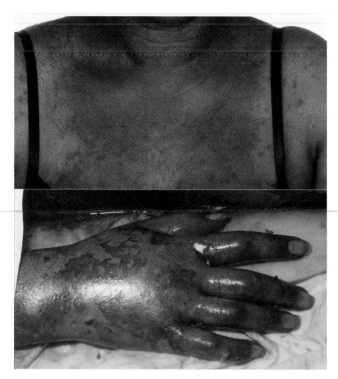

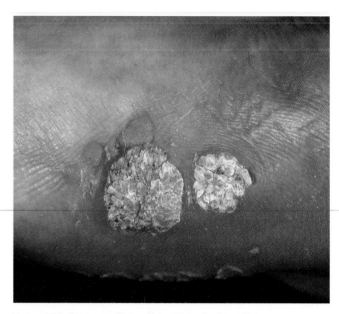

**Figure 14.6** Human papilloma viral warts on the foot. Discrete hyperkeratotic nodules with a rough, filiform surface.

**Figure 14.5** Drug rashes. Photosensitive eruption on the chest due to St. John's Wort, widespread skin sloughing secondary to toxic epidermal necrolysis due to nevirapine.

alongside systemic symptoms. The HLA-B*5701 allele is associated with a significantly increased risk of a hypersensitivity reaction to abacavir and pre-screening is recommended. Other drug rashes in HIV patients include mucosal ulceration (zalcitabine, foscarnet), phototoxic rashes (St John's Wort) (Figure 14.5), Stevens–Johnson syndrome (cotrimoxazole, nevirapine and efavirenz) and toxic epidermal necrolysis (TEN) (nevirapine, abacavir, cotrimoxazole). TEN is 1000 times more common in HIV-positive individuals, and is characterized by painful, rapid, widespread (>30% of skin surface area) full thickness skin necrosis (Figure 14.5) associated with a 25–30% risk of mortality.

## Human papillomavirus (HPV)

Approximately 20–30% of HIV patients are affected by HPV infections. Mucosal infections may be latent (DNA detection), subclinical (detected by 3–5% acetic acid application) or clinical. Cutaneous lesions are readily apparent, often multiple, clustered, widespread and occasionally profuse (Figure 14.6). Multiple plane warts may be seen as a marker of occult HIV disease. Anogenital disease (condylomata acuminata) is characterized by exophytic verrucous lesions that may become cancerous. Deep plantar warts can be painful and usually contain 'black specks' which are thrombosed capillaries. Skin warts have a heterogeneous appearance including hyperkeratotic papules, nodules, small plaques, filiform and mosaic lesions.

The diagnosis is clinical; however, cytology and DNA subtyping may be helpful. Cutaneous warts are moderately resistant to treatment in the context of HIV. However, salicylic and lactic acid can

be effective at high concentrations if used regularly. A course of cryotherapy (liquid nitrogen) can be efficacious but may be painful, and transient blistering can result. Curettage and cautery may be performed but causes scarring and there is a risk of recurrence. Immunotherapies such as imiquimod and diphencyprone can be used, but the results are often disappointing.

## Molluscum contagiosum

Molluscum contagiosum is caused by pox virus, commonly seen in HIV patients particularly in the beard area (Figure 14.7). The lesions are usually flesh-coloured papules with umbilicated centres; however, atypical forms are also reported. Hundreds of small mollusca are often present and occasionally very large lesions arise

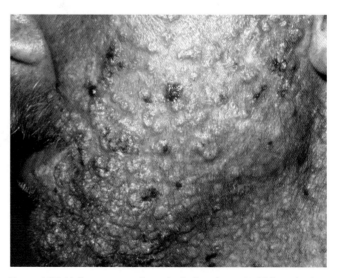

**Figure 14.7** Molluscum contagiosum in the beard area. Multiple coalescing umbilicated shiny papules.

(giant mollusca). Molluscum lesions tend to persist in HIV patients, resulting in significant cosmetic embarrassment. The diagnosis is usually a clinical one; however, a smear from the central keratotic plug or skin biopsy reveals multiple characteristic molluscum inclusion bodies. Initiation of cART can cause mollusca lesions to undergo spontaneous regression or paradoxically worsen initially. Persistent lesions can be treated with cryotherapy (10–15 seconds per mollusca) or cautery after topical anaesthesia (EMLA). Giant lesions may only respond to curettage. Topical imiquimod 5% or cidofovir may be effective for resistant lesions.

### Herpes simplex virus

Herpes simplex virus (HSV)-1 and HSV-2 commonly cause infections in HIV patients, with 60–80% of patients co-infected with HSV-2. The frequency and duration of HSV infections rises with CD4 counts <50 cells/μL. Deteriorating ulceration (Figure 14.8) however can occur after the commencement of cART, due to the reconstitution of the patients' immune system, so-called immune reconstitution syndrome (IRS). Commonly affected sites are the anogenital and perioral regions. Acute lesions are characterized by vesicles which progress to crusted, eroded and eventually 'punched-out' ulcerated lesions that may become chronic. Recurrent ulceration may lead to giant ulcers (10–20 cm). HSV isolation by cell culture, electron microscopy or immunofluorescence studies on lesional fluid taken by scrapings or swabs. Polymerase chain reaction availability is increasing and is a rapid, highly reproducible, method of HSV detection. Aciclovir treatment is given for localized HSV infections; the dose in HIV patients is usually 400 mg five times a day for 5–10 days. If aciclovir is ineffective, consider resistant HSV (absent viral thymidine kinase) and change to foscarnet 40 mg/kg iv tds, or vidarabine 15 mg/kg iv daily. Valacyclovir has been shown to be superior to famciclovir in the suppression of HSV-2 reactivation.

### Candidiasis

*Candida* yeast infections have a predilection for mucous membranes and warm moist skin flexures. Oral candidiasis (thrush) classically presents with white plaques on a background of inflammation, but in chronic infections there may be persistent glossitis and cobblestone mucosae. Oropharyngeal infections may spread locally to the oesophagus in HIV patients. Flexural *Candida* is characterized by erythema with peripheral satellite lesions (Figure 14.9). Swabs for microscopy and culture may isolate the yeast. Superficial *Candida* infections can be treated with topical antifungals including clotrimazole, miconazole and nystatin in several formulations including lozenges, oral gel, pessaries, and creams. Refractory disease requires systemic therapy with fluconazole 100 mg or itraconazole 200 mg daily for 2 weeks.

### Tinea infections

Cutaneous fungal infections of the body (corporis), groin (cruris), feet (pedis) and scalp (capitis) are common in immunosuppressed patients, and are often extensive. Lesions are usually itchy.

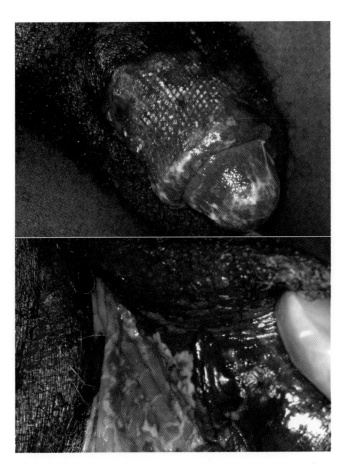

**Figure 14.8** Herpes simplex virus. Extensive genital ulceration associated with immune reconstitution syndrome.

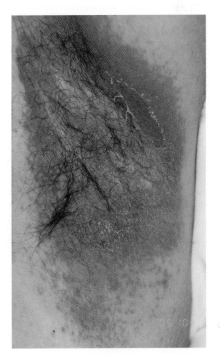

**Figure 14.9** Candida in the axilla. Confluent macerated erythema with peripheral satellite lesions.

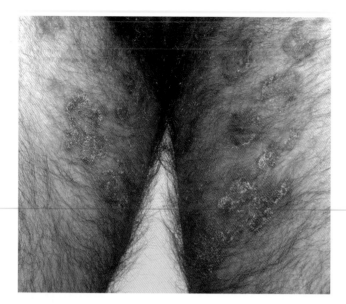

**Figure 14.10** Tinea cruris. Annular erythematous scaly eruption in the groin.

Annular erythematous plaques with a raised scaly edge may be seen (Figure 14.10). Clinical features may be significantly altered by topical steroids (tinea incognito). Mycological scrapings may isolate the fungus. First-line topical treatment is terbinafine 1% cream twice daily for 2–4 weeks; alternatives are miconazole and ketoconazole. Itraconazole 100 mg for 2 weeks is an effective systemic therapy. Fluconazole 150 mg once weekly for 2–4 weeks. Terbinafine 250 mg daily for 4 weeks is used to treat tinea capitis infections.

## Scabies

*Sarcoptes scabiei* mite infestation is common in HIV patients and is usually transmitted by close personal contact. Intractable itching disturbs sleep. Patients present with itchy papules especially on the flanks, axillae and genitals, occasionally burrows are seen (finger webs, genitals). HIV patients may develop crusted scabies, which is highly contagious, and characterized by hyperkeratotic papules and plaques (Figure 14.11). Secondary skin changes such as eczema and impetigo may occur. Microscopy from a burrow scraping or crust can confirm the presence of mites. Scabies in the context of HIV can be difficult to eradicate. First-line treatment is 5% permethrin cream to all skin surfaces from the neck downwards, left on for 12 hours. The treatment should be repeated after 1 week. All close personal contacts should be treated simultaneously. Bedding, towels and underclothing should be washed. Systemic ivermectin is the preferred treatment for crusted scabies and recalcitrant infestations.

## Syphilis

The World Health Organization estimates the number of new cases of syphilis worldwide each year to be around 12 million. Co-infection of syphilis with HIV in the USA and Europe is reported to be between 20% and 70%. The presentation of syphilis in HIV patients may be atypical, but classically a painless genital ulcer develops 3–4 weeks after transmission. Secondary syphilis presents with a rash, fever, arthralgia and lymphadenopathy 4–8 weeks after the primary infection. The rash characteristically affects the trunk, palms and soles (Figure 14.12) and is non-pruritic. Early lesions are usually annular erythematous macules that fade to a greyish-brown. Serological testing for syphilis should be performed to confirm the diagnosis. Primary/secondary syphilis should be treated with a single dose of i.m. benzathine penicillin 2.4 mega units, or i.m. procaine penicillin 600 000 units daily for 10 days. Latent syphilis requires longer treatment.

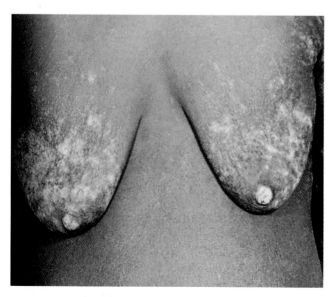

**Figure 14.11** Crusted scabies. Confluent crusting and scaling over the chest.

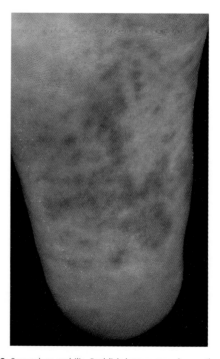

**Figure 14.12** Secondary syphilis. Reddish-brown macules on the sole of the foot.

**Table 14.1**  Common dermatological manifestations of HIV infection.

| Skin condition | CD4 count (cells/uL) | Typical distribution | Morphology of lesions/rash | Symptoms |
|---|---|---|---|---|
| Seborrhoeic dermatitis | Particularly <100 | Scalp, eyebrows, nasal creases, chest | Greasy scales with underlying eczema | Mild pruritus |
| Pruritic papular eruption | Particularly <250 | Trunk, neck and face | Excoriated follicular papules | Intense pruritus |
| Nodular prurigo | Any | Limbs, trunk | Excoriated firm nodules | Intense pruritus |
| Scabies | Any | Fingerwebs, genitals, trunk | Burrows, excoriated papules, crusting | Intense pruritus keeps patient awake at night |
| Human papilloma virus | Any | Face, fingers, feet, genitals | Hyperkeratotic papules | None |
| Molluscum contagiosum | Any | Face, arms, groin | Umbilicated flesh coloured papules | None |
| Kaposi sarcoma | Particularly <200 | Mouth, face, perineum | Violaceous macules, patches, nodules | None |

## Penicillium marneffei, Cryptococcus neoformans, Histoplasma capsulatum

These opportunistic fungal infections usually affect HIV patients with a CD4 count of less than 50 cells/μL. Patients infected with *Penicillium marneffei* are usually unwell with non-specific fever, lymphadenopathy and hepatosplenomegaly, two-thirds of patients have multiple umbilicated papules and nodules on their skin that mimic molluscum contagiosum. Skin biopsy for histology and culture is diagnostic in 90% of cases. Only 10% of patients infected with *Cryptococcus neoformans* develop skin lesions; these are similar to the umbilicated nodules seen in *Penicillium* infections; however, ulcers and/or pinpoint haemorrhages (petechiae) may also occur. *Histoplasma capsulatum* infections are mainly characterized by respiratory disease. Skin lesions may manifest as erythema nodosum or erythema multiforme; however, with dissemination multiple pustules and nodules can appear on the skin containing the fungus.

## Conclusions

Skin conditions in HIV-infected populations are common and varied. In order to confirm the diagnosis a number of tests could be performed, including syphilis serology, skin scraping and viral PCR. Skin biopsy is an important tool in the armament of a clinician attempting to diagnose a dermatological condition (Table 14.1).

## Further reading

Eisman S. Pruritic popular eruption in HIV. *Dermatol Clin* 2006;24:449–457.

Gottschalk GM. Paediatric HIV/AIDS and the skin: an update. *Dermatol Clin* 2006;24:531–536.

Hogan MT. Cutaneous infections associated with HIV/AIDS. *Dermatol Clin* 2006;24:473–495.

Honda KS. HIV and skin cancer. *Dermatol Clin* 2006;24:521–530.

Martins CR. Cutaneous drug reactions associated with newer antiretroviral agents. *J Drugs Dermatol* 2006;5:976–982.

# CHAPTER 15

# The Kidney and HIV

*J. Booth and J. Connolly*

UCL Centre for Nephrology, Royal Free Hospital, London, UK

## OVERVIEW

- Acute renal failure remains common in the HIV population, usually due to pre-renal causes, acute tubular necrosis or drug injury
- Chronic kidney disease is a growing problem as patients with HIV live longer; causes are both specific to HIV e.g. HIV-associated nephropathy or more general e.g. hypertension
- All patients with HIV should be screened for kidney disease by urinalysis for protein and measurement of estimated glomerular filtration rate
- Antiretroviral drugs should be dosed according to renal function, and some, e.g. nucleotide reverse transcriptase inhibitors, have serious renal adverse effects that require monitoring
- Haemodialysis and renal transplantation are now being used with increasing success in end-stage renal disease in HIV

## Introduction

The dramatically improved patient survival afforded by combination antiretroviral therapy (cART) has served to unmask chronic kidney disease as a major determinant of health in the HIV population. Up to 30% of patients with HIV show evidence of chronic kidney disease (Table 15.1) with either proteinuria on urinalysis or an elevated serum creatinine, and these abnormalities are associated with an increased risk of death.

Effective treatment for HIV has also led to a shift in the spectrum of renal diseases affecting those with HIV, and while conditions such as HIV-associated nephropathy (HIVAN) remain important, new problems such as the renal toxicity of antiretroviral drugs have also emerged.

This chapter focuses on the important renal disorders encountered in HIV along with approaches to their diagnosis and management.

## Evaluating renal disease in HIV

The finding of an elevated serum creatinine or abnormalities of urine dipstick are often the first pointers towards the presence

of renal disease in HIV. A targeted history should follow to seek the presence of urinary symptoms, pain or oedema, relevant drug exposures, including cART, and pointers towards the presence of hypovolaemia (e.g. diarrhoea). Blood pressure should be checked and volume status assessed clinically.

Urine dipstick will detect the presence of protein, blood or glucose, whereas microscopy may show red cell casts, suggesting glomerulonephritis. Protein levels should be quantified by measuring a urinary protein–creatinine ratio, a spot urine measurement that correlates well with formal 24-hour measurements of protein excretion.

When taken alone, serum creatinine is a poor indicator of the absolute glomerular filtration rate (GFR) as baseline levels vary widely between patients of differing age, sex or race (Figure 15.1). Various equations have been developed that incorporate such variables to give a more accurate prediction of GFR (so-called estimated or eGFR) and the four-variable modification of diet in renal disease (MDRD) formula is preferred in the UK. Chronic kidney disease has recently been reclassified into five stages of severity on the basis of eGFR. Caution should be exercised when interpreting eGFR in patients with HIV in whom wide variation in muscle mass or the use or creatine or protein supplementation may make the MDRD equation inaccurate.

**Table 15.1** Classification of chronic kidney disease according to estimated glomerular filtration rate (eGFR, mL/min/1.73 m$^2$).

| Stage | Description |
|---|---|
| 1 | eGFR >90* <br> Normal GFR |
| 2 | eGFR 60–90* <br> Mild renal impairment |
| 3 | eGFR 30–60 <br> Moderate renal impairment <br> Frequently asymptomatic |
| 4 | eGFR 15–30 <br> Severe renal impairment <br> Anaemia, bone disease, fluid, electrolyte and acid-base disturbances common |
| 5 | eGFR <15 <br> Established renal failure. Impending need for renal replacement therapy |

*Stages 1 and 2 only apply if other evidence of kidney disease exists, e.g. structural abnormality or persistent proteinuria.

*ABC of HIV and AIDS*, Sixth Edition. Edited by Michael W. Adler, Simon G. Edwards, Robert F. Miller, Gulshan Sethi and Ian G. Williams.
© 2012 Blackwell Publishing Ltd. Published 2012 by Blackwell Publishing Ltd.

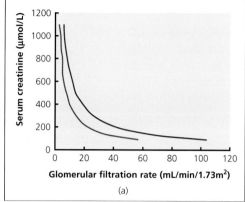

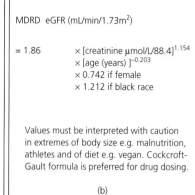

**Figure 15.1** (a) Relationship between serum creatinine and glomerular filtration rate. Purple line – 30-year-old Afro-Caribbean man. Blue line – 70-year-old Caucasian woman. Note the large difference in GFR for similar serum creatinine values. (b) Four-variable Modification of Diet in Renal Disease (MDRD) formula for calculation of estimated glomerular filtration rate.

Ultrasound of the renal tract will exclude obstruction and may also point to specific pathology, for instance the enlarged echogenic kidneys often seen with HIVAN. Renal biopsy is frequently required to make a definitive diagnosis in cases where the results of non-invasive tests alone are insufficient.

## Acute renal failure

Episodes of acute renal failure are common in the HIV population, the majority due either to pre-renal causes, such as hypovolaemia or severe sepsis, or intrinsic renal events. The latter include ischaemic acute tubular necrosis, drug injury and less common causes such as rhabdomyolysis and haemolytic-uraemic syndrome. Opportunistic infection is a common setting for acute renal failure in HIV, both due to severity of illness and the array of potentially nephrotoxic antimicrobials used in treatment (Table 15.2).

Episodes of acute renal failure can generally be managed conservatively with appropriate volume resuscitation and removal of nephrotoxic agents. Treatment should also be directed at the underlying cause where necessary, e.g. opportunistic infection.

**Table 15.2** Common nephrotoxins encountered in the care of patients with HIV.

| Drug | Renal adverse effect |
| --- | --- |
| **Antibiotics** | |
| Co-trimoxazole | ATN, acute TIN, hyperkalaemia |
| Aminoglycosides e.g. gentamicin | ATN |
| Sulfadiazine | Crystalluria, haematuria and nephrolithiasis |
| **Antivirals** | |
| Aciclovir | Crystallisation with tubular obstruction |
| Foscarnet | ATN, glomerulonephritis, RTA |
| **Antifungals** | |
| Amphotericin | ATN, proximal tubular dysfunction |
| **Antiretrovirals** | |
| Indinavir, atazanavir | Nephrolithiasis, chronic TIN |
| NtRTIs, e.g. tenofovir | Proximal tubular dysfunction |
| NRTIs, e.g. didanosine | Lactic acidosis |

Co-trimoxazole, trimothoprim–sulfamethoxazole; ATN, acute tubular necrosis; TIN, tubulointerstitial nephritis; RTA, renal tubular acidosis.

Complications such as hyperkalaemia, acidosis and fluid overload should be monitored for and temporary recourse to renal replacement may be required in the most severe cases.

## HIV-associated nephropathy

Rao and colleagues first described a syndrome of heavy proteinuria with rapidly progressive renal failure among the AIDS population of New York in 1984. Histological appearances, with focal and segmental glomerulosclerosis and marked interstitial nephritis, appeared to resemble heroin nephropathy, but many patients had no history of intravenous drug abuse. Subsequent case series emphasized the frequent and striking histological finding of collapse of the glomerular tuft. In the years to follow, HIV-1 has been intimately linked to the pathogenesis of this condition, which has become known as HIV-associated nephropathy (HIVAN).

HIVAN is the most common cause of end-stage renal disease in HIV, and is almost exclusively seen in people of Afro-Caribbean or Hispanic ethnicity. The prevalence within the African American HIV population is estimated at 3.5–12%. Classically considered a late manifestation of HIV infection, recent evidence suggests that HIVAN may also occur earlier in the course of infection when immune responses are well maintained.

### Pathogenesis

HIVAN results from direct infection of renal tissue by the HIV virus although host factors play an important role in expression of disease. Infection of podocytes results in severe cellular dysregulation, with dedifferentiation and proliferation. Podocyte foot processes are lost, which culminates in collapse of the capillary loop producing the typical histological lesion. Animal studies have suggested an important role for the HIV accessory gene *nef* in initiating these events. Recent studies have confirmed a genetic association with MYH9 and APOL1 genes in African-Americans with HIVAN.

### Clinical features

HIVAN is characterized clinically by nephrotic-range proteinuria and marked renal impairment. Despite significant hypoalbuminaemia, patients frequently have little oedema and are often normo- or hypotensive. Ultrasound of the renal tract often reveals enlarged, echogenic kidneys. Renal biopsy is required to confirm the diagnosis.

Histological findings are of focal and segmental glomerulosclerosis, mesangial hyperplasia and variable collapse of the glomerular tuft as the glomerular basement membrane pulls away from the visceral epithelium. Renal tubular atrophy with microcystic dilatation is also seen. Immunostaining of tissue is often negative and characteristic tubuloreticular inclusions are seen within glomerular endothelial cells on electron microscopy.

## Treatment

Without intervention, HIVAN progresses rapidly towards end-stage renal disease over weeks to months. cART appears to prolong renal survival and forms the current backbone of treatment. The current recommendation is to commence cART at the time of HIVAN diagnosis, irrespective of the CD4 count or stage of disease. Maximal benefit is obtained if virus is kept persistently suppressed.

Blood pressure should be tightly controlled to a target of 125/75 using angiotensin converting enzyme inhibitors or angiotensin receptor blockers (ARBs). Older data from small non-randomized studies suggest corticosteroids may improve renal function and slow disease progression but this has not been confirmed and steroids are now rarely used.

## Immune complex kidney disease

Immune complex-mediated glomerular diseases constitute as much as three-quarters of all chronic kidney disease in HIV. Patterns of disease include those unique to HIV, such as HIV immune complex kidney disease (HIVICK), and those which are also prevalent in the general population, e.g. membranous glomerulonephritis, IgA nephropathy. Immune complexes formed between antibody and HIV antigens such as p24 have been detected in the kidneys of HIV-infected patients with glomerulonephritis and are postulated to be pathogenic. Presenting features include proteinuria, haematuria and renal impairment, but diagnosis requires renal biopsy as differentiation from HIVAN is usually not possible on clinical grounds alone.

HIVICK describes a unique histological pattern of mesangial and subepithelial immune deposits that produce a characteristic 'ball in cup' appearance on light and electron microscopy. Immunofluorescence shows variable staining of deposits for IgA, IgM, IgG and C3.

Few organized clinical trials have addressed the treatment of immune complex disease in HIV. Small retrospective studies have produced conflicting data on the efficacy of cART in this setting. Most clinicians choose to initiate cART on diagnosis, as this seems rational if HIV accounts for the immune dysregulation causing the disease. Case reports support the efficacy of corticosteroids, but their use is limited by the increased risk of infection.

## Antiretroviral drugs and the kidney

cART has revolutionized HIV care but at the expense of a broad range of adverse effects. Although many antiretrovirals have been linked in case reports to renal adverse events, it is the drugs indinavir, tenofovir and atazanavir that have received most attention. A large European cohort analysis showed that these three drugs were associated with an increased risk of developing chronic kidney disease for each year of exposure. Careful monitoring for renal toxicity is required for individuals taking HIV medication (Table 15.2).

## Tenofovir

Tenofovir is an acyclic nucleotide reverse transcriptase inhibitor (NtRTI) and is excreted unchanged in the urine. Initial prospective trials with tenofovir showed no evidence of nephrotoxicity, but since becoming widely available in clinical practice more than 50 reports have been published linking tenofovir to the development of Fanconi syndrome.

Fanconi syndrome is characterized by the triad of normoglycaemic glycosuria, hypophosphataemia and tubular proteinuria and is underpinned by a failure of reabsorptive mechanisms in the proximal tubule (Figure 15.2). Symptoms may include lethargy, polyuria, polydipsia and severe muscular weakness. Osteomalacia, on occasions severe, may develop as a result of prolonged hypophosphataemia. A rise in creatinine is an insensitive marker of the Fanconi syndrome and usually occurs late in disease.

The finding of glycosuria with a normal plasma glucose, hypophosphataemia and proteinuria (generally less than 2 g per 24 hours) in a patient receiving tenofovir are highly suggestive of Fanconi syndrome and should prompt discontinuation of the drug. Where necessary renal biopsy will exclude most alternative pathologies, and may show the typical tubular cell changes of thinning and vacuolation. The biochemical abnormalities associated with tenofovir toxicity usually resolve completely within 1–2 months after treatment is discontinued.

## Indinavir

Nephrolithiasis has been reported to occur with all ritonavir-boosted protease inhibitors but none more so that indinavir. Indeed, it is the renal complications of indinavir which have led to it rarely being used in the UK.

Indinavir is excreted in the urine after metabolism by the liver, where it has a tendency to precipitate at pH values above 4.5 and form rectangular plate or fan-shaped crystals. Sludging of crystalline aggregates within the renal tract can lead to flank pain, haematuria and dysuria as well as classical renal colic. A provoking factor, such as dehydration is often present. Microscopic cystalluria is present in up to 65% of patients, but the majority remain asymptomatic. The stones are radiolucent and thus not visible on plain radiographs. Renal tract ultrasound or CT imaging is required for diagnosis.

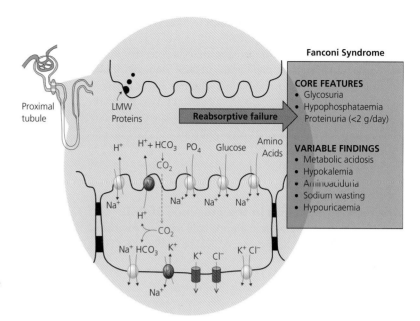

**Figure 15.2** The Fanconi syndrome results from reabsorptive failure in the proximal tubule. LMW, low molecular weight; $PO_4$, phosphate; $HCO_3$, bicarbonate.

Indinavir therapy has also been linked with insidious loss of renal function in the absence of urological symptoms or evidence of renal obstruction. Biopsy typically reveals a tubulointerstitial nephritis with marked fibrosis and evidence of crystals within the distal tubules. Improvement in renal function is variable after stopping treatment. This pattern of renal impairment appears to be associated with a persistent leucocyturia on urinalysis, and periodic monitoring of urine for white cells and serum creatinine is recommended in the first 6 months of indinavir treatment, with biannual checks thereafter.

### Atazanavir

Cases of renal stones linked with atazanavir have been reported and the drug has been confirmed to be present in the stones using infrared spectroscopy.

### Renal monitoring in HIV infection

Careful monitoring is important to detect renal toxicity at an early stage (Table 15.3). A baseline urinalysis, serum phosphate and renal function should be obtained at diagnosis and prior to starting treatment, and these parameters should then be checked regularly thereafter. More frequent monitoring is recommended if other risk factors for chronic kidney disease (CKD) are present or the patient is taking nephrotoxic drugs. Ideally, proteinuria should be assessed by formal measurement of urine protein creatinine ratio as dipstick analysis detects primarily albuminuria and is insensitive for the low molecular weight proteinuria characteristic of tenofovir toxicity.

**Table 15.3** Recommendations for monitoring of patients receiving the anti-retroviral medications indinavir and tenofovir.

| Drug | Recommendations |
|---|---|
| Tenofovir | Urinalysis (for glucose or protein), serum calcium, phosphate and creatinine pre-treatment |
| | Periodic (optimum frequency) checks for development of glycosuria, proteinuria, or hypophosphataemia; Fanconi syndrome may not develop until months or years after starting tenofovir. |
| | Increased surveillance if: |
| | Receiving a ritonavir-boosted protease inhibitor; pre-existing renal impairment; diabetic or hypertensive; receiving other potential nephrotoxic medications e.g. aciclovir; older age e.g. >50 years |
| Indinavir | Urinalysis (for leucocytes and blood) and serum creatinine pre-treatment |
| | Periodic urinalysis and serum creatinine during first 6 months; twice per year thereafter |
| | Patients to drink 1.5L water per day to reduce chance of stone formation |

### Renal replacement therapy

Survival rates for HIV-positive individuals with end-stage renal disease now rival the general population. Haemodialysis and peritoneal dialysis are both viable options for renal replacement in HIV, although the former tends to be preferred. Native arteriovenous fistulae are preferred to artificial grafts or tunnelled lines for haemodialysis access as the infection and thrombosis rates are significantly lower. Dialysis units operate strict infection control protocols, minimizing any risk of transmission to other patients.

Renal transplantation has the potential to transform the quality of life and improve survival of patients with end-stage renal disease but until recently was considered contraindicated in HIV due to the burden of exogenous immunosuppression required. Studies now suggest that with careful patient selection and planning of immunosuppression regimens, graft and patient survival rivals the general population for both cadaveric and live-related transplants. Patients must have an HIV viral load of <50 copies/mL for 6 months with good adherence to a stable antiretroviral regimen in order to be considered, with no active infections or AIDS-defining illnesses.

### Antiretroviral dosing in the presence of CKD

Dose alteration of nucleoside and nucleotide reverse transcriptase therapy is required in the presence of mild to moderate CKD: no adjustment is usually required for other antiretroviral agents. Careful consideration of dosing of all HIV drugs is required during renal replacement therapy and the use of therapeutic drug monitoring may be required.

## Further reading

EACS guidelines http://www.europeanaidsclinicalsociety.org/images/stories/EACS-Pdf/eacsguidelines-v6_english.pdf.

IDSA. Guidelines for the Management of CKD in HIV Infected Individuals. (www.idsociety.org/assets/0/18/312/924/D35A41AB-4B98-4314-A57D-0A3C339B719A.pdf).

# CHAPTER 16

# Sexually Transmitted Infections and HIV

*P. French*

Mortimer Market Centre, London, UK

**OVERVIEW**

- HIV is predominantly a sexually transmitted infection (STI)
- STIs facilitate the transmission of HIV
- People with STIs or at risk of STIs should have HIV testing
- People with HIV should have ongoing STI risk assessment and STI testing
- The diagnosis and treatment of STIs in HIV-positive individuals is usually straightforward

There is a close and complex relationship between HIV infection and other sexually transmitted infections (STIs). HIV is predominantly sexually transmitted and shares the same behavioural risk factors as other STIs. STIs facilitate the transmission of HIV and HIV may alter the natural history of other STIs. Some oncogenic viruses which can predispose HIV-positive individuals to serious ill health (HHV8, Epstein–Barr virus and human papilloma virus (HPV) 16, hepatitis B and hepatitis C) may be or are usually sexually transmitted (see Chapters 7 and 11). In addition to this, most individuals with HIV are at risk of STI acquisition after HIV diagnosis, making STI care an important part of the ongoing care for many people with HIV.

## HIV as an STI

HIV is usually an STI, with the major routes of transmission being vaginal and anal sex. As it shares many of the risk factors associated with the acquisition of other STIs, HIV testing should be recommended to all patients presenting for STI testing and care, especially those in whom another STI has been diagnosed.

## STIs as a cofactor in HIV transmission

STIs are an important co-factor in the transmission of HIV. This is particularly infections associated with genital inflammation – cervicitis, urethritis and proctitis (gonorrhoea, chlamydia, lymphoganuloma venereum (LGV)), vaginitis (trichomoniasis)

and genital ulcer disease (particularly syphilis, herpes simplex and chancroid). A variety of mechanisms explain this association. Susceptibility to HIV is increased when there is a loss of mucosal/epithelial barriers. There is also an increased number of CD4 lymphocytes and other targets of HIV in inflamed epithelial tissues. Loss of normal vaginal flora and a reduction in the acidity of vaginal fluid (as occurs in bacterial vaginosis) may also contribute to the increased susceptibility of women to HIV.

The risk of sexual transmission is proportional to the HIV viral load in genital secretions, and cell-associated and cell-free HIV is increased in the presence of genital inflammation. The increase in HIV viral load in genital secretions associated with STIs decreases when STIs are treated. This was first described in seminal fluid after the treatment of urethritis but has now been noted in cervicitis and genital ulcer disease.

Table 16.1 gives summary of the relative risk of increased susceptibility of HIV acquisition in the presence of STIs.

A considerable proportion of HIV transmission is attributable to the presence of STIs, making STI control one of the cornerstones of HIV control programmes. An important community randomized study of enhanced STI treatment in Mwanza, Tanzania, showed a 40% reduction in HIV incidence in communities where STI treatment and care had been strengthened. In addition to this, STI treatment and care should be part of the care of all those with HIV.

## HIV and STI co-infection

Individuals diagnosed with HIV remain at risk of STI acquisition, and there have recently been STI outbreaks among men who have

**Table 16.1** The relative risk for HIV susceptibility for different sexually transmitted infections (STIs)/genital infections.

| STI | Effect estimate (relative risk) | 95% confidence interval |
|---|---|---|
| Any STI | 3.7 | 2.7–5.0 |
| *Trichomonas vaginalis* – women only | 1.5 | 1.2–2.0 |
| Gonorrhoea | 2.1 | 1.7–2.5 |
| Chlamydia | 2.2 | 1.4–3.3 |
| Syphilis | 2.5 | 2.1–3.1 |
| Chancroid | 2.1 | 1.2–3.4 |
| Bacterial vaginosis – women only | 1.4 | 1.0–2.0 |

Adapted from Røttingen *et al.* (2001).

*ABC of HIV and AIDS*, Sixth Edition. Edited by Michael W. Adler,
Simon G. Edwards, Robert F. Miller, Gulshan Sethi and Ian G. Williams.
© 2012 Blackwell Publishing Ltd. Published 2012 by Blackwell Publishing Ltd.

sex with men (MSM) that have disproportionately affected HIV positive MSM. Since the late 1990s there have been outbreaks of syphilis, sexually acquired hepatitis C and anorectal lymphogranuloma venereum among MSM in Europe, North America and Australia. A large proportion of these men were co-infected with HIV, and these outbreaks appear to be predominantly related to behavioural risks rather than a biological increase in susceptibility to infection. Key features of these outbreaks are noted in Box 16.1.

> **Box 16.1 Features of STIs/HIV outbreaks**
>
> - Syphilis – oral sex is an important transmission route
> - Lymphogranuloma venereum (LGV) – anorectal syndrome (inguinal syndrome rare)
> - Hepatitis C (HCV) – associated with unprotected (without a condom) anal intercourse
> - All outbreaks associated with HIV-positive MSM
> - Concomitant STIs common. LGV may predispose to sexual acquisition of HCV

However, HIV may increase the risk of STI acquisition. Longitudinal studies of female commercial sex workers in Africa have shown an association between increasing HIV-associated immunosuppression and the prevalence of chancroid, genital herpes, syphilis and trichomoniasis, suggesting a causal link.

The presentation, diagnosis and treatment of STIs in individuals with or without HIV are usually identical (see *ABC of Sexually Transmitted Infections*) but can be modified, particularly in individuals who are severely immunocompromised. Possible differences in presentation and management of some STIs are outlined below and summarized in Boxes 16.2 and 16.3.

> **Box 16.2 Syphilis – Differences in Presentation of syphilis in HIV positive vs HIV negative**
>
> - Primary syphilis – larger, multiple, painful ulcers
> - Secondary syphilis – genital ulcers, higher titre RPR/VDRL
> - Neurosyphilis – higher risk of asymptomatic neurosyphilis, possibly higher risk and quicker progression to symptomatic neurosyphilis

> **Box 16.3 Differences in natural history of STIs in HIV positive vs HIV negative individuals**
>
> - Genital herpes* – larger, chronic ulcers, increase in asymptomatic shedding
> - Genital warts* – larger, recalcitrant exophytic warts
> - Chancroid – multiple, atypical ulcers
> - Pelvic inflammatory disease – severe presentation (fever and possibly tubo-ovarian abscess more common)
>
> *Oral warts and exophytic herpes may complicate immune reconstitution after the initiation of cART.

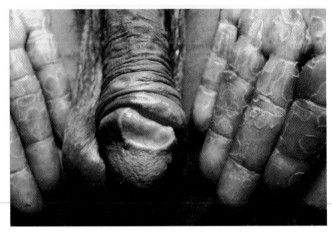

**Figure 16.1** Concomitant primary syphilis (genital ulcer) and secondary syphilis (palmar rash). Photo courtesy of Professor D. Mabey.

## Bacterial STIs
### Syphilis (Box 16.2)

HIV-positive individuals with early syphilis are more likely to present with larger, multiple and painful ulcers in primary syphilis and to have genital ulceration as a feature of secondary syphilis (Figure 16.1). In addition the RPR/VDRL diagnostic tests (markers of disease activity) tend to be lower in primary syphilis and overall are higher in secondary syphilis. The extent to which HIV impacts on the progression of syphilis to later stages of syphilis, particularly neurosyphilis, is controversial. Some studies have noted more frequent central nervous system involvement in early syphilis and a number of case reports suggest a more rapid disease progression. Undoubtedly neurosyphilis must be part of the differential diagnosis of all HIV-positive patients with neurological syndromes.

### Chancroid

Ulcers due to chancroid may be larger and more likely to be multiple in HIV-positive individuals. Some studies suggest that ulcers may be slower to heal but other studies have shown that treatment response is unrelated to HIV status.

### Pelvic inflammatory disease

There is some evidence that HIV-positive women with chlamydia are more likely to subsequently develop pelvic inflammatory disease (PID) than HIV-negative women with chlamydia. Although women with HIV may present with more severe PID, the response to standard therapy appears to be unrelated to HIV status.

## Viral STIs
### Herpes simplex infection

As HIV disease progresses genital herpes episodes tend to become more frequent, more extensive and longer. There is also an increased risk of asymptomatic shedding, which combined with increases in episode frequency significantly increase the risk of onward transmission of herpes. Patients with severe immunosuppression may

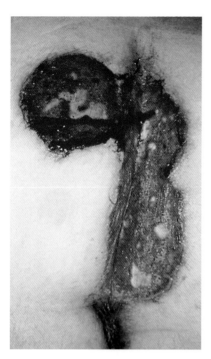

**Figure 16.2** Large chronic erosive perianal ulceration due to herpes virus.

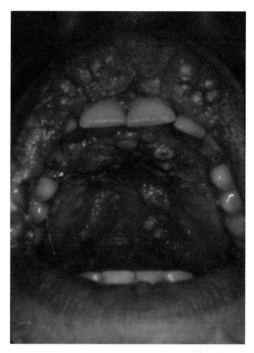

**Figure 16.3** Mouth warts associated with HIV immune reconstitution. Photo courtesy of Professor J. Zakrewska.

develop atypical chronic erosive and slowly progressive ulceration (Figure 16.2). This usually settles well with aciclovir (valaciclovir or famciclovir are equally efficacious) but there is a risk of the development of antiviral resistance in this situation. The best treatment for this syndrome is reversal of immunosuppression with combination antiretroviral therapy (cART).

Commencement of cART can be occasionally associated with the emergence of raised (exophytic) herpes simplex, but this usually responds to aciclovir (or valaciclovir/famciclovir).

### Genital warts

Recalcitrant genital warts can be a problem associated with HIV immunosuppression but usually respond well to standard therapy and reconstitution of the immune system with cART.

However, emergence of warts for the first time (especially oral warts) is a well-recognized feature of immune reconstitution (Figure 16.3).

### Oncogenic HPV

The sexually acquired subclinical oncogenic HPVs (especially HPV 16 and 18) continue to be important pathogens in HIV-infected individuals, even in parts of the world where cART is available.

All women with HIV should have regular screening for cervical intraepithelial neoplasia (CIN) and treatment of CIN if it is identified to prevent the development of cervical cancer.

There is increasing evidence of a link between the presence of HPV 16, the development of anal intraepithelial neoplasia and the subsequent development of anal carcinoma (see Chapter 7). However, it remains uncertain whether enough is known about the natural history of this condition or the effectiveness of proposed interventions to prevent the progression of AIN to recommend routine screening for AIN at present.

## Diagnosis and management of STIs

The close association of HIV and other STIs means that it is important for people with HIV to have STI care available to them, and increasingly HIV treatment and care services are offering STI care as a routine part of healthcare.

People with HIV have many ongoing sexual healthcare needs, which means that STI care should be integrated with other sexual healthcare, including sexual health promotion, condom provision, pre-conception advice, fertility control and post-exposure prophylaxis for HIV exposure for HIV-negative partners. A number of models have been suggested for this and a summary of the STI recommendations from the British HIV Association/British Association for Sexual Health and HIV are in Box 16.4.

---

Box 16.4 **Models of sexual healthcare**

BASHH/BHIVA Recommended standards for sexual healthcare of people with HIV (2008)

- Women – yearly cervical cytology
- Hepatitis B and C serology – yearly testing if still at risk
- Syphilis testing – three monthly
- Full STI screen – yearly
- Sexual risk assessment – 6 monthly

The diagnosis and treatment of STIs are usually straightforward and a number of regularly updated national and international guidelines are available online (see Box 16.5).

---

Box 16.5 **National/International STI treatment guidelines**

- CDC (USA), www.cdc.gov/std/treatment/2010/
- WHO Guideline, www.who.int/hiv/pub/sti/pub6/en/index.html
- IUSTI (European), www.iusti.org/regions/europe/euroguidelines.htm
- BASHH (UK), www.bashh.org/guidelines

---

## Further reading

Fakoya A, Lamba H, Mackie N, *et al.* BHIVA, BASHH and FSRH Standards for the management of the sexual and reproductive health of people living with HIV infection 2008. *HIV Medicine* 2008,9:681–720.

Grosskurth H, Mosha F, Todd J, *et al.* Impact of improved treatment of sexually transmitted diseases on HIV infection in rural Tanzania: randomised controlled trial. *Lancet* 1995;346:530–536.

Rogstad K (ed.) *ABC of Sexually Transmitted Infections*, sixth edition. BMJ Books, 2011.

Røttingen, J-A, Cameron WD, Garnett, GP. A systematic review of the epidemiological interactions between classic sexually transmitted diseases and HIV: how much really is known? *STDs* 2001;28:579–597.

# CHAPTER 17

# Women and HIV

*C. Wilkinson and D. Mercey*

Central and North West London NHS Foundation Trust, London, UK

## OVERVIEW

- The natural history and overall management of HIV in women does not differ significantly from that in men
- For optimum outcome of a pregnancy in an HIV-positive mother, an experienced multidisciplinary team should be involved from diagnosis
- With correct management almost all mother-to-child transmission of HIV can be prevented
- No method of contraception is contraindicated solely on the basis of a woman being HIV infected, with the exception of vaginal barriers used with spermicide
- The most effective method of emergency contraception is a copper intrauterine device
- The efficacy of many forms of contraception (including emergency contraception) can be affected by combination antiretroviral therapy
- Sperm washing and artificial insemination are examples of interventions that can help minimize transmission of HIV in discordant couples who are trying to conceive

## Psycho-social issues

The diagnosis of HIV infection may be devastating for any individual and lead to anxiety, depression and stress; however, there may be additional considerations for newly diagnosed women who may have to consider the possible HIV-positive status of any children and the implications for future pregnancies. Women may fear, or actually experience, violence from their partner on disclosure of their status. As carers some women may find it difficult to prioritize their own health needs.

## Natural history

The natural history of HIV infection is not significantly different between men and women when the mode of acquisition of HIV is controlled for. A similar spectrum of opportunistic infection

*ABC of HIV and AIDS*, Sixth Edition. Edited by Michael W. Adler,
Simon G. Edwards, Robert F. Miller, Gulshan Sethi and Ian G. Williams.
© 2012 Blackwell Publishing Ltd. Published 2012 by Blackwell Publishing Ltd.

and malignancy is seen, and guidelines for antiretroviral treatment suggest using similar CD4 cut offs for deciding when to start therapy. The same antiretroviral drugs are used, except that women at risk of, or planning, a pregnancy should avoid the use of potential teratogens. Response to therapy does not appear to differ significantly between men and women.

## Pregnancy management in the developed world

As policy in much of the developed world including the UK is to recommend an HIV test as part of all women's antenatal care, and as women with diagnosed HIV are now remaining well for longer, more women with HIV are being managed in pregnancy. For women who are first diagnosed HIV-positive during pregnancy, it is important to recognize that this may present complex issues for the patient regarding disclosure of her status to partner and family. Help with multiple psychosocial issues such as adjustment to the diagnosis, immigration and housing may be required. The issue of testing other children as well as her partner must also be addressed.

There is a small risk that some women may acquire HIV during pregnancy. Consideration should be given to repeat HIV testing in women who may be at higher risk of HIV acquisition and those who present with typical HIV seroconversion-like symptoms. National guidance (BHIVA, 2008) also recommends near patient bedside testing for HIV for untested women in labour.

For women with diagnosed HIV infection who plan to become pregnant, it is important to optimize their HIV treatment and review the need for any regular medication they may be taking. An STI screen is advised and should be repeated during the pregnancy.

The management of HIV-positive pregnant women should be undertaken by a multidisciplinary team to include, as a minimum, a specialist midwife, an HIV specialist, an obstetrician and a paediatrician, but others may need to be involved (Box 17.1). The health of a woman who is well at the outset of pregnancy is probably not compromised by an uncomplicated pregnancy and the likelihood of an adverse pregnancy outcome is only slightly greater than in the general population, with the possible exception of a greater risk of early preterm delivery.

Without intervention, a breastfeeding mother has a 20–30% risk of transmission of HIV to her baby. This can be reduced to approximately 1% by the use of antiretrovirals, avoidance of breastfeeding and caesarean section in certain situations. For women who are not on therapy and who do not require therapy for their own health they may choose between

- zidovudine monotherapy with a caesarean section if their viral load is consistently below 10 000
- short-course combination therapy starting after the first trimester with an option of a vaginal delivery if an undetectable viral load is achieved.

A resistance assay is recommended before treatment is started and should be repeated after treatment is discontinued.

Women who require treatment for their own health should be treated with combination antiretroviral therapy (cART), starting as soon as practicable. Reports to date do not suggest any excess of fetal abnormalities in babies exposed to antiretrovirals *in utero*, with the possible exception of didanosine. Up-to-date information about pregnancy outcomes is available through the Antiretroviral Pregnancy Register (www.apregistry.com). Maternal toxicity from antiretroviral drugs is well recognized and advice should be sought from an experienced HIV clinician before commencing therapy in pregnancy. British and European guidelines on the management of HIV infection in pregnancy are regularly updated and available online for up to date advice on specific HIV therapies.

Women who conceive while taking combination therapy should continue this if it is well tolerated and achieving an undetectable viral load. No antiretroviral medications are licensed for use in the first trimester. The unknown long and short term effects of conceiving on cART should be discussed. Where therapy is failing, the woman presents late in pregnancy or presents with threatened premature delivery, specialist advice should be sought.

Studies showing that an elective caesarean section reduces the risk of transmission from mother to child were conducted before the routine use of cART so the additional benefit of caesarean section in these women is not known. Women who achieve and

maintain an undetectable viral load on combination therapy may elect to have a vaginal delivery.

All babies born to HIV-positive women should be given 4 weeks of antiretroviral treatment, usually with a monotherapy component of the maternal treatment. Combination treatment may be required where the baby was delivered to a mother on combination therapy with a detectable viral load, suggesting poor adherence or resistance and for babies whose mothers received no cART.

All babies should be formula fed to reduce the risk of HIV transmission associated with breastfeeding.

Parents should be advised that the HIV status of their baby can be confirmed by PCR testing by 3 months of age. Follow-up for all infants exposed to antiretrovirals *in utero* or born to an HIV-positive mother should be arranged.

## Pregnancy management in the developing world

It is not possible to generalize care guidelines to the whole of the developing world as access to components of optimal therapy vary greatly. However, all women should have access to HIV testing during pregnancy, with the option of at least short course cART to minimize HIV transmission to their babies. Recent data from Botswana (www.nejm.org/doi/full/10.1056/NEJMoa0907736) has shown that the risk of HIV transmission to babies in women who initiate cART during pregnancy and continue throughout breastfeeding is 1.1%. Avoidance of breastfeeding is not possible unless access to safe and sustainable supplies of formula feed can be arranged, and even then bottle feeding may not be acceptable because of the implied HIV-positive status. Owing to these considerations the World Health Organization recommends that HIV-positive mothers or their infants take antiretrovirals while breastfeeding to prevent HIV transmission.

## Gynaecological care

For the most part, the gynaecological care of women with HIV is similar to that provided to women without HIV/AIDS, the main exceptions being in relation to fertility treatment, cervical cancer prevention and genital infections such as human papilloma virus (HPV), herpes simplex virus (HSV) and *Candida*, which are more likely to be recurrent or severe.

### Cervical screening

HIV infection increases the risk of both cervical cancer and cervical intraepithelial neoplasia (CIN) and appears to be associated with immunosuppression. CIN is present in between 20% and 40% of women with HIV.

All women newly diagnosed with HIV and who are aged 25 years or over should have cervical screening if not performed within the last 12 months. Some recommend baseline colposcopy due to the prevalence of false-negative smear results, but this is dependent on resources. Thereafter, annual cytology should be performed with referral for colposcopy based on UK national guidelines. High-grade

CIN (2 and 3) should be managed according to national guidelines. However, recurrences are common, reportedly being as high as 80% in women with CD4 counts below 200 cells/μL. Low-grade lesions should not usually be treated as they probably represent persistence of HPV infection, which responds poorly to treatment. Regular cytological monitoring is mandatory.

cART appears to increase the regression of low-grade lesions. However, the effect on high-grade lesions and HPV persistence is less clear and women on cART should be managed as other HIV-positive women.

## Genital infections

Women with HIV may experience genital infections such as herpes simplex, candidiasis or warts that are more severe, recurrent or persistent than in women without HIV infection. For the most part the treatment regimens are unaltered, but prophylactic or specialist referral may be required (Table 17.1).

## Contraception

Women requesting contraception, including those with HIV, should be supported to make an informed choice of the most effective method that is acceptable to them (Box 17.2). The role of healthcare providers is to ensure safe choice and support effective use. Efficacy between methods varies. Long-acting reversible contraceptives (LARC) (Figure 17.1) are the most effective reversible methods (Table 17.2), and are comparable to permanent methods such as female and male sterilization; however, the latter is the most effective method.

With the exception of vaginal barriers (caps and diaphragms), which require nonoxynol-9 use, all methods are suitable for most women. The UKMEC (Table 17.2) provides basic guidance on the

| Box 17.2 **Information to be provided to women requesting contraception** |
| :--- |
| • Typical use failure rates |
| • Principal side effects, and known risks |
| • Non-contraceptive benefits, e.g. reduction of menorrhagia or amenorrhoea |
| • Use and follow-up (including advice on drug interactions and use of emergency contraception and duration of use) |
| • Use of condoms in addition to another method to prevent transmission of HIV |

use of contraception with medical conditions. Care is needed in the UKMEC in women with multiple conditions. Depo-Provera (DMPA) has been associated with reduced bone mineral density (BMD), although not osteoporosis and fracture; caution should be exercised in women at risk of reduced BMD and other methods considered. Drug interactions are important; hepatic enzyme-inducing drugs, including some cART, are likely to reduce the efficacy

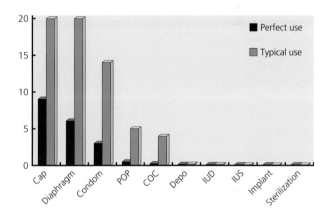

**Figure 17.1** Contraceptive failure rates (%) in first year of use demonstrating the difference between methods and perfect and typical use. Adapted from the CG-30 Clinical Guideline on Long Acting Contraception. NICE 2005.

**Table 17.1** Treatment regimens.

| Diagnosis | Single episode treatment | Treatment or persistence or frequent recurrence |
| :--- | :--- | :--- |
| Herpes simplex | 5–7 days duration, may be extended in severe infections<br>○ Treatment aciclovir 200 mg 5 × a day orally<br>or<br>○ Valaciclovir 500 mg twice daily<br>or<br>○ Famciclovir 250 mg three times daily<br>If oral therapy not appropriate aciclovir 5–10 mg/kg 8 hourly iv | If recurrences frequent and episodic oral treatment may be prescribed to be initiated by the patient early in a recurrence<br>Prophylaxis (at least 6 episodes per annum)<br>Aciclovir 400 mg 2 × day. Discontinued after 1 year to assess recurrences, but good data on long-term safety |
| Genital candidiasis | Topical or systemic anti-fungal agents (e.g. clotrimazole, fluconazole) | Systemic antifungals (oral imidazoles) are sometimes used long term to prevent recurrence. |
| Genital warts | Topical therapy (podophyllotoxin or imiquimod) or cryotherapy | Refer if not responding to treatment |

**Table 17.2** UK contraceptive medical eligibility criteria for women with HIV.

| | COC | POP | DMPA | Implant | IUD | IUS | Condom | Diaphragm |
| :--- | :--- | :--- | :--- | :--- | :--- | :--- | :--- | :--- |
| High risk of HIV | 1 | 1 | 1 | 1 | 2 | 2 | 1 | 3 |
| HIV positive, not using cART | 1 | 1 | 1 | 1 | 2 | 2 | 1 | 3 |
| HIV positive, using ART | 1–3* | 1–3* | 1-2* | 1-2* | 2 | 2† | 1 | 3 |
| AIDS using ART | 2* | 2* | 2 | 2* | 2 | 2 | 1 | 3 |

1 = no restriction for use of the method.
2 = the advantages of using the method generally outweigh the theoretical or proven risks.
3 = the theoretical or proven risks generally outweigh the advantages of using the method.
4 = method should not be used due to unacceptable health risk.

*Some cARTs may interact with contraceptive steroids and reduce the efficacy of the method.
†Although a low dose progestogen-only method available evidence suggests no loss of efficacy when used concomitantly with hepatic enzyme inducers.

of combined oral contraceptives (COCs), progestogen only pill (POP) and implants and should not be used without condoms and after considering all other methods. DMPA (Depo-Provera), IUS (intrauterine system) and IUD (intrauterine device) are not known to be affected by liver enzyme inducers. Consistent condom use should be encouraged in conjunction with other methods.

## Emergency contraception

Women should be advised of the indications for emergency contraception (EC) and how to access it. A copper IUD is the most effective method and can be used within 5 days of intercourse, and importantly depending on the menstrual history often beyond this. Progestogen-only emergency contraception (POEC) containing levonorgestrel is available without prescription in the UK or from a healthcare provider and is best used as early as possible within 72 hours of intercourse. A new prescription-only oral emergency contraceptive, ulipristal acetate (UA), a selective progesterone receptor modulator, is now licensed for use up to 120 hours after intercourse in the UK. Available evidence suggests that this is more effective than POEC, but it can be used only once in a cycle, and because of its mechanism of action may reduce the efficacy of hormonal contraceptives started immediately after taking UA. Women on hepatic enzyme-inducing drugs should consider an IUD or double the dose of POEC, which is off-licence and of unknown efficacy, there is no guidance on the use of UA in these patients. The use of UA is not recommended in women using medication that increases gastric pH.

## Subfertility

Discordant couples without established subfertility require advice to minimize HIV transmission risk. Sperm washing is the treatment of choice where the man is HIV positive and should carry no risk of transmission. However, for some couples timed unprotected intercourse may be the only accessible treatment, which carries a risk of transmission. HIV-positive women can use self-insemination and should be provided with information on doing this. For those with established subfertility many investigations can be carried out in primary care but those requiring assisted conception should be referred to a specialist unit experienced at providing care for couples with HIV.

## Further reading

BASHH. Guidelines on Diagnosis and Management of STI. (www.bashh.org).

BHIVA. Guidelines for the Management of HIV Infection in Pregnant Women and the Prevention of Mother-to-Child Transmission of HIV. (www.bhiva.org).

EACS (www.europeanaidsclinicalsociety.org/guidelinespdf/EAEuroGuidelines_FullVersion.pdf).

FSRH. Guidelines on use of contraceptive methods, including emergency contraception are available from www.fsrh.org.

NICE. Clinical guideline on Long Acting Reversible Methods of Contraception. 2005 (www.nice.org.uk).

UK Selected Medical Eligibility Criteria for contraceptive use (2009). FSRH. www.fsrh.org Management of sexual and reproductive health of people living with HIV infection (2007). BHIVA, FFPRHC, BASHH. 2007 www.bhiva.org.

# CHAPTER 18

# HIV Infection in Children

*P. McMaster[1] and S. Stokes[2]*

[1]North Manchester General Hospital, Manchester, UK
[2]Emergency Medicine Trainee, Oxfordshire Deanery, UK

---

**OVERVIEW**

- The success of prevention of mother to child transmission has resulted in numbers of children with HIV plateauing globally and infections in newborns are now rare in the UK

- Exclusive breastfeeding is recommended where there is a high mortality from gastroenteritis with maternal combination antiretroviral therapy, but strongly discouraged in industrialized countries.

- Testing for HIV is the most important step that any health professional can do without the need for specialist counselling

- Supportive care is essential to motivate adolescents to adhere to treatment

---

## Epidemiology

### International

Worldwide, approximately 1000 children under 15 years old are infected every day. An estimated 270 000 children die each year from an HIV-related cause. Over 90% of the children with HIV in the world live in Sub-Saharan Africa. In parts of KwaZulu Natal more than one-third of pregnant women have HIV infection. Owing to expanded access to combination antiretroviral therapy (cART) in progress the rate of new infections in children in Africa has decreased since a peak in 2001. However, in parts of Asia it is still increasing. Young people age 15–24 years account for 45% of all new HIV infections in adults, with 2800 new infections every day in 18–24 year olds (Figure 18.1).

### UK and Ireland

A total of 1704 children with HIV have been reported to the Collaborative HIV Paediatric Study (CHIPS), a cohort study of all HIV-infected children in the UK and Ireland, to March 2011. Of those in current follow-up ($n = 1190$), 79% are of black African ethnicity, and virtually all are infected through mother-to-child transmission. Previously the majority were seen in clinics in London; however, the dispersal of asylum seekers country-wide

means there are now as many elsewhere in the UK, and numbers in London have plateaued. The rate of hospital admissions has decreased throughout the last decade, and there have been fewer than 10 deaths per year since 2005. Around 300 to date have transferred to adult clinics (Figure 18.2).

## Prevention of mother-to-child transmission

Effective control of HIV during pregnancy using cART alongside avoidance of breastfeeding has the ability to almost eliminate mother-to-child transmission of HIV infection. In low- to middle-income countries the challenge has been making the required antiretrovirals (ARVs) accessible to pregnant women. The World Health Organisation (WHO) policy had been to balance affordability with practicality using single doses of ARVs. However, this placed the mother at risk of HIV drug resistance and did not provide protection of transmission following delivery where breastfeeding is a recommended baby feeding strategy. WHO now recommends earlier initiation of cART for adults and adolescents and prolonged use of treatment to reduce the risk of mother-to-child transmission. The Joint United Nations Programme on HIV/AIDS (UNAIDS) is committed to a goal of eliminating new paediatric HIV infections by 2015. It recommends that countries adopt a policy of either HIV-positive mothers or their infants take cART while breastfeeding to prevent HIV transmission (Table 18.1).

### Breastfeeding

With no interventions, 15–20% of infants born to mothers with HIV will be infected through breastfeeding for 18–24 months. However, this has to be balanced against the risk of death through gastroenteritis and its sequelae. There are several factors that should be taken into account in balancing the risks of replacement feeding against the risk of HIV transmission (Box 18.1 AFASS criteria). Where these factors outweigh the risks of transmission, reducing the maternal viral load to undetectable levels with cART offers the best current solution, without totally removing the risk of infection. Where clean water is accessible, replacement feeds are advised. Challenges remain such as the cost of formula for low-income families, and the stigma of replacement feeding, which may indicate the mother's HIV status by proxy.

---

*ABC of HIV and AIDS*, Sixth Edition. Edited by Michael W. Adler,
Simon G. Edwards, Robert F. Miller, Gulshan Sethi and Ian G. Williams.
© 2012 Blackwell Publishing Ltd. Published 2012 by Blackwell Publishing Ltd.

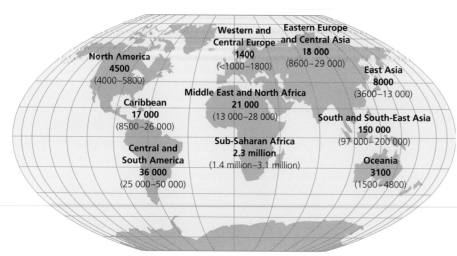

**Total: 2.5 million** (1.6 million–3.4 million)

**Figure 18.1** Children (<15 years) estimated to be living with HIV 2009: UNAIDS. Reproduced with permission from UNAIDS.

Box 18.1 **AFASS criteria**

Acceptable: The mother perceives no problem in replacement feeding. Potential problems may be cultural, social, or due to fear of stigma and discrimination.

Feasible: The mother (or family) has adequate time, knowledge, skills, resources and support to correctly mix formula or milk and feed the infant up to 12 times in 24 hours.

Affordable: The mother and family, with community or health system support if necessary, can pay the cost of replacement feeding without harming the health or nutrition status of the family.

Sustainable: Availability of a continuous supply of all ingredients needed for safe replacement feeding for up to one year of age or longer.

Safe: Replacement foods are correctly and hygienically prepared and stored, and fed preferably by cup.

*Source:* IMCI Complementary Course on HIV/AIDS; Module 3; Counselling the HIV Positive Mother. WHO 2007.

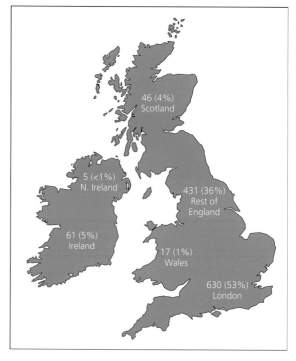

**Figure 18.2** Regional distribution of main follow-up clinic for 1190 children alive and followed up in CHIPS. Children who have died, lost to follow-up, left the UK and Ireland or transferred to adult care are excluded.
*Source:* Reproduced with permission of Collaborative HIV Paediatric Study (CHIPS).

## Testing

The first step in managing HIV and reducing its transmission is the diagnosis of infection. Before combined ARVs were available, the ethical issues of testing were more challenging, and voluntary counselling and testing were emphasized. At that stage HIV became stigmatized because of high mortality and its label as a sexually transmitted disease. However, now there is much greater emphasis on 'routine' HIV testing undertaken by health professionals with no specific training in HIV counselling. The outstanding issue with regard to paediatric testing surrounds establishing a timetable for the earliest possible diagnosis, before the child becomes immuno-compromised, while supporting parents through the process. In infancy there is greater urgency to test because of the risk of rapid progression of disease, and even in older children if the parents have not voluntarily agreed to testing within 6 months the child protection team should involve social services.

Infants of infected mothers require testing for the virus with PCR until maternal antibodies have cleared, which may take 2 years. In the UK the routine is to test at birth, 6 weeks and 3 months.

The reduction in mother-to-child transmission means that there are fewer newly infected children and there are more children who were vertically infected now entering adulthood. Many of these will be long-term non-progressors who maintain good CD4 counts well into the second decade without any symptoms. The importance of this is that the 'children' of infected mothers should be tested no matter what age they are, how well they are or when the mother thinks she may have been infected unless there is evidence of a neg-ative test after delivery or completing breastfeeding. Post-exposure prophylaxis may also require testing to be repeated up to 3 months

**Table 18.1** Mother-to-child transmission rates.

| Intervention | Transmission rates | Reference studies |
|---|---|---|
| No intervention | 32% | UNAIDS reference group on estimates, modelling and projections |
| No intervention; long breastfeeding (BF) | 35% | De Cock review, 2000 |
| No intervention 6-month BF | 30% | De Cock review, 2000; DITRAME: RETRO-CI, 1999 |
| Replacement feeding (RF) | 20% | De Cock review, 2000; Bangkok CDC, 1999 |
| Single dose (SD) NVP mother and infant, 6-month BF | 16% | HIVNET 012, 2003 |
| SD NVP, RF | 11% | SAINT NVP, 2003 |
| AZT from 28 weeks, SD NVP, 6-month BF | 10% | DITRAME plus, 2005 |
| AZT from 28 weeks, SD NVP, RF | 2% | Thai PHPT-2, 2004 |
| cART, AZT 4 weeks infant, RF | 0.7% | NSHPC, 2011 |
| cART, AZT 4 weeks infant, RF, Caesarean section | 0.7% | NHSPC, 2011 |

later, although newer 4th generation assays are usually positive by 6 weeks (Figure 18.3).

## Management

### Clinical features

The greatest risk of life-threatening opportunistic infections occurs in infancy. Cytomegalovirus (CMV) and *Pneumocystis jiroveci* (previously *carinii*) can produce overwhelming respiratory failure from the first month of life (Figure 18.4). Untreated, gastroenteritis and sepsis are common causes of death during the first year. The HIV virus can also cause an encephalopathy, ranging from a severe spastic quadriplegia to more insidious developmental or psychological impairment. Other indications for testing for HIV include recurrent upper respiratory tract infections, lymphadenopathy, hepato/splenomegaly, dermatitis or parotitis. Markers of more advanced disease (Centers for Disease Control category B or WHO Clinical Stage 2 or 3) include anaemia, neutropenia or thrombocytopenia; pneumonia, bacteraemia, oral candidiasis, recurrent or

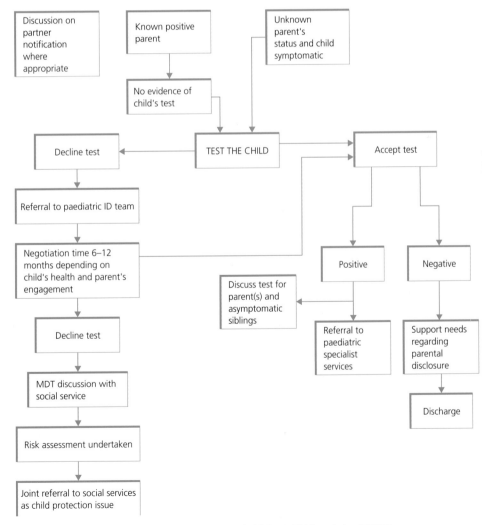

**Figure 18.3** Don't forget the children. *Source:* Reproduced with permission of Children's HIV Association (CHIVA).

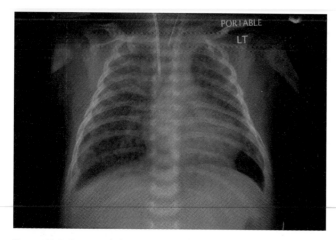

**Figure 18.4** Cytomegalovirus pneumonitis in 2-month-old infant.

chronic diarrhoea, herpes stomatitis and persistent or complicated varicella. CDC category C or WHO Stage 4 are AIDS defining (Figure 18.4).

## Monitoring

Once a diagnosis of HIV is made, infants under 1 year old should be started on treatment as soon as possible. Older children need to be followed up to assess three factors in terms of when to start treatment: (1) CD4 count; (2) clinical status; and (3) social factors. CD4 counts are high in infancy but drop to near adult levels by about 6 years of age. Under this age the percentage of CD4 to total lymphocytes is a useful guide (see PENTA (Paediatric European Network for the Treatment of AIDS) guidelines Table 18.2). Clinical features of advanced disease such as developing increasing lymphadenopathy, hepatosplenomegaly, dermatitis, faltering growth and episodes of infections are used as a guide for treatment initiation. The main purpose of treatment is to raise the CD4 count and prevent opportunistic infections. However, these decisions are balanced against the risk of developing resistance through lapses in adherence and the adverse effects of ARVs (Table 18.2).

## Antiretrovirals

There is extensive experience in children of use of the three main classes of ARVs: nucleoside/nucleotide reverse transcriptase inhibitors (NRTIs), non-nucleoside reverse transcriptase inhibitors (NNRTIs) and protease inhibitors (PIs). There is little but growing use of integrase inhibitors in children (e.g. raltegravir) but limited experience of entry inhibitors (e.g. maraviroc – CCR5 inhibitor). The first joint study between the main European and US paediatric

**Table 18.2** PENTA guidelines for when to start cART.

| Age (years) | CD4 count (cells/μL) | CD4% | Clinical |
|---|---|---|---|
| <1 | Treat all | | |
| 1–3 | <1000 | <25% | If > 1 year and symptomatic* |
| 3-5 | <500 | <20% | If symptomatic* |
| >5 | <350 | – | If symptomatic* |

*CDC stage B or C / WHO stage 3 or 4.

HIV trials groups, PENPACT 1, showed equivalent outcomes in those children given NNRTI or PI-based therapy. The usual policy of two NRTIs and an NNRTI or a PI is sometimes modified depending on resistance and adherence using other combinations or PI monotherapy. There are combination tablets with two NRTIs and nevirapine with paediatric doses produced in India but not licensed in UK. The choices of cARTs will be based on resistance profiles as well as social issues such as preferences for once- or twice-daily regimens (Table 18.3).

## Resistance

The HIV virus is an RNA virus that replicates by integration into host DNA. This process results in frequent errors in the copied amino acids. Some of these mutations result in resistance to ARVs. Infants may be infected with both fully susceptible 'wild-type' virus and resistant virus from the mother. This may happen either at the same time, usually at delivery, or sequentially, for example from breastfeeding. Resistant virus usually replicates less effectively than wild type and so when an infant is tested for mutations off-treatment it may show no mutations, but it is important to look at previous resistance tests in the mother to look for archived virus. Likewise

**Table 18.3** Antiretroviral formulations.

| | UK license | Liquid formulation |
|---|---|---|
| **NRTI** | | |
| Lamivudine | >3 months | Yes |
| Abacavir | >3 months | Yes |
| Zidovudine | All ages | Yes |
| Emtricitabine | >4 months | Yes |
| Didanosine EC | >6 years | No |
| Stavudine | >3 months | Yes |
| Tenofovir DF | Not children | |
| **NNRTI** | | |
| Neviripine | >50 kg | Yes |
| Neviripine prolonged release | >3 years | |
| Efavirenz | >3 years | Yes |
| Etravirine | Not children | |
| Rilpivirine | Not children | |
| **PI** | | |
| Kaletra (lopinavir/ritonavir) | >2 years | Yes |
| Darunavir | Not first line | No |
| Atazanavir | ≥6 years | No |
| Ritonavir | ≥2 years | Yes |
| Saquinavir | Not children | No |
| Fosamprenavir | ≥6 years | Yes |
| Tipranavir | 2-12 years | Yes |
| Nelfinavir | >3 years | No |
| **Fusion inhibitor** | | |
| Maraviroc | Not children | No |
| **Integrase inhibitor** | | |
| Raltegravir | Not children | No |
| **Co-formulations** | | |
| Kivexa | Weight dependent | No |
| Truvada | Weight dependent | No |
| Atripla | Weight dependent | No |
| Eviplera | Not children | |

NRTI, nucleoside/nucleotide reverse transcriptase inhibitor; NNRTI, non-nucleoside reverse transcriptase inhibitors; PI, protease inhibitor.

**Table 18.4** Guidelines for the use of ARVs in Paediatric HIV Infection.

**First-line antiretroviral therapy**

| <3 years | >3 years but <40 kg | >40 kg |
| --- | --- | --- |
| NVP + 3TC + ABC (+ AZT) | EFV + 3TC + ABC | EFV + (FTC + TDF) or EFV +(3TC + ABC) |
| or | or | or |
| LPV/r + 3TC + ABC (+ AZT) | LPV/r + 3TC + ABC | LPV/r + (FTC + TDF) or LPV/r + (3TC + ABC) |

**Most likely second-line combined antiretroviral therapy – when first-line NNRTI based**

| <30 kg | >30 kg | >40 kg |
| --- | --- | --- |
| LPV/r + AZT + DDI | LPV/r + AZT + TDF | Previous (FTC + TDF) →LPV/r + DDI + ABC<br>Previous (3TC + ABC) →LPV/r + AZT + TDF |

**Most likely second-line combined antiretroviral therapy – when first line PI based**

| <3 years | >3 years but <30 kg | >30 kg | >40 kg |
| --- | --- | --- | --- |
| NVP + AZT + DDI | EFV + AZT + DDI | EFV + AZT + TDF | Previous (FTC + TDF) →EFV + DDI + ABC<br>Previous (3TC + ABC) →EFV + AZT + TDF |

ABC, abacavir; AZT, zidovudine; DDI, didanosine; EFV, efavirenz; LPV/r, Kaletra; NVP, nevirapine; TDF, tenofovir; 3TC, lamivudine.
*Source:* Paediatric European Network for Treatment of AIDS 2009 Guidelines. http://www.chiva.org.uk/files/guidelines/PENTA2009.pdf.

the choice of ARVs for prevention of mother-to-child transmission should be determined by previous maternal resistance tests. When adherence is poor, it is safer to stop treatment while support is given before restarting when there is greater confidence that the treatment will be taken (Table 18.4).

### Adherence

One of the greatest challenges for treating young people is avoiding the development of resistance to ARVs. The decision of which medicine to choose will be tailored to suit the child's age and risk of poor adherence. Some of the tablets/capsules are large and due to limited dose ranges may need to be cut or dissolved in water. A challenging issue for young children is finding ARVs in a palatable liquid form that are stable at room temperature. However, some syrups such as Kaletra have an unpleasant taste and as the child grows the volume of liquid becomes an issue. There are few choices of ARVs, and mutations often make the virus resistant to all drugs in a class. Adherence to medication regimens in adults is an informed choice, but with children it is a child protection issue. Tools, like pill boxes with alarms or automated text messages, can improve adherence in adolescents but most important is education and peer support (Figure 18.5).

### Adverse effects

ARV medication toxicities are better reported in adults than in children. The older NRTIs such as stavudine and didanosine were more prone to causing lipodystrophy in adults. As children grow and body shape changes both lipoatrophy and changes in fat distribution can go unrecognized for longer. Immediate adverse effects of nausea and diarrhoea cause problems with adherence, although in the majority this settles in the first couple of weeks. Young people are often concerned that their peers will ask about the mild jaundice associated with atazanavir. Renal toxicity of tenofovir is seen in childhood but is reversible if detected early by urine protein to creatinine ratio. The impact in children of certain drug toxicities that are commonplace in adults such as cardiovascular disease and osteoporosis is unknown.

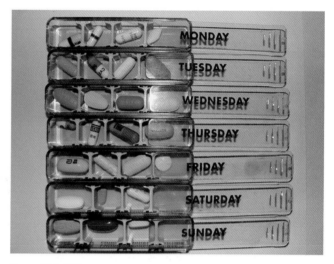

**Figure 18.5** Pill box.

### Transition

Of the children with HIV in the UK and Ireland, the proportion aged 10 years and over increased from 11% in 1996 to 70% in 2010. Adolescence is a difficult time of adjustment from parent-led supervision of treatment to independence in all areas of life. The unique difference with antiretroviral treatment is that the typical non-adherence to treatment can mean life-long viral resistance after missing very few doses (probability increases the more doses missed). The most successful key to adherence seems to be motivating the young person from an early age to accept responsibility for their treatment with decreasing supervision. This is achieved by providing the education they require for understanding the condition and how the medicines work. Paediatricians are also challenged to expand their usual comfort zone of history taking to allow young people to feel at ease talking about sex, alcohol and drug use. When care is finally transferred to adult services, joint 'transition' clinics are vital to avoid omissions in follow-up and maintain trust between the patient and healthcare professionals (Figure 18.6).

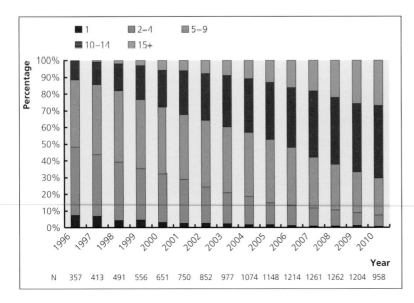

**Figure 18.6** Age distribution of children with HIV in UK 1996–2010. Age is taken to be age at start of the year or age at presentation if child presented during that year. Data are for children and young people receiving paediatric care; those who have transferred to adult clinics are not included. *Source:* Reproduced with permission of Collaborative HIV Paediatric Study (CHIPS).

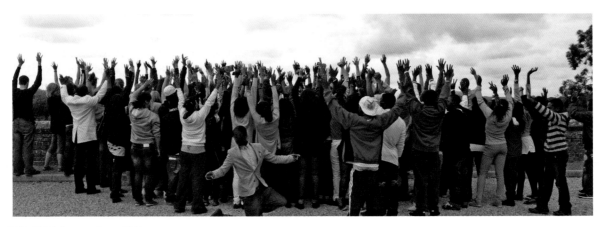

**Figure 18.7** CHIVA Support Camp 2010.

## Supportive care

The key to success in HIV management in children is providing appropriate support throughout childhood. When a mother is diagnosed, the paediatric team should be involved in preparing the family for testing and neonatal prophylaxis and providing support for them coming to terms with the possibility that they could have infected their child. Continued intense support is required for medication adherence in younger children and promoting independence and trust among more mature children. The stigma associated with HIV often prevents disclosure in school but the role of voluntary sector organizations is essential to give young people the opportunity to talk to their peers in a safe environment at social events or summer camp (Figure 18.7).

## Further reading

Babiker A, Castro nee Green H, Compagnucci A, *et al.* (study team). First-line antiretroviral therapy with a protease inhibitor versus non-nucleoside reverse transcriptase inhibitor and switch at higher versus low viral load in HIV-infected children: an open-label, randomised phase 2/3 trial. PENPACT-1 (PENTA 9/PACTG 390. *Lancet Infect Dis* 2011;11:273–283.

CHIVA. Don't Forget the Children. (www.chiva.org.uk/files/repository/pdf/dont-forget-children.pdf).

Judd A, Doerholt K, Tookey PA, *et al.* Morbidity, mortality, and response to treatment by children in the United Kingdom. Collaborative HIV Paediatric Study. *Clin Infect Dis* 2007;45:918–924 (www.chipscohort.ac.uk).

PENTA 2009 guidelines for the use of antiretroviral therapy in paediatric HIV-1 infection. *HIV Med* 2009;10:591–613 (www.pentatrials.org).

UNAIDS. *UNAIDS Report on the Global AIDS Epidemic 2010.* (www.unaids.org/globalreport).

# CHAPTER 19

# Antiretroviral Drugs

*P. Benn[1], G. Sethi[2] and I. G. Williams[3]*

[1] Mortimer Market Centre, London, UK
[2] Guy's and St Thomas' Hospital, London, UK
[3] University College London Medical School, London, UK

## OVERVIEW

- There are more than 25 different drugs within six classes which interfere with the HIV life cycle
- First-line treatment should include three antiretroviral agents, which usually consists of two nucleoside/tide analogues and either a non-nucleoside or a protease inhibitor as the third agent. This is often referred to as highly active antiretroviral therapy (HAART) or combination antiretroviral therapy (cART).
- Life-long continuous treatment is recommended, as intermittent therapy has been shown to be associated with increased rates of complications (HIV and non HIV)
- Resistance testing is recommended prior to starting treatment due to the risk that patients may have acquired, or developed, drug-resistant virus
- Co-formulations of drugs commonly used to treat HIV infection have helped to reduce pill burden and improve adherence
- The choice, tolerability and clinical effectiveness of cART has improved markedly over the last decade. This has led to guidelines recommending earlier initiation of therapy

Since 1996 in the developed world there have been dramatic falls in the incidence of new AIDS cases and AIDS-associated deaths. Published data in the late 1990s estimated the mortality rate in patients with CD4 counts of less than $100 \times 10^6$/L had fallen by nearly two-thirds to <8 per 100 person years. Although the long-term clinical efficacy of the current antiretroviral treatment regimens remains uncertain, the biological rationale for maintaining a clinical response has been established. Sustained inhibition of viral replication results in partial reconstitution of the immune system in most patients, substantially reducing the risk of clinical disease progression and death. Strategies to sustain suppression of viral replication in the long term will be necessary. There are several potential targets for antiretroviral drugs in the viral replication cycle (Figure 19.1). Six classes of antiretroviral drugs are currently licensed for use in combination for the treatment of HIV infection. Once initiated, life-long continuous treatment is recommended as intermittent therapy has been shown to be associated with increased

*ABC of HIV and AIDS*, Sixth Edition. Edited by Michael W. Adler,
Simon G. Edwards, Robert F. Miller, Gulshan Sethi and Ian G. Williams.
© 2012 Blackwell Publishing Ltd. Published 2012 by Blackwell Publishing Ltd.

rates of HIV and non-HIV disease complications. New therapeutic agents and treatment strategies are constantly being evaluated.

## Reverse transcriptase inhibitors

The first drugs made available for clinical use were inhibitors of the HIV reverse transcriptase. Before the virus can be integrated into the host cell genome DNA, a copy of the viral RNA has to be formed (proviral DNA). This is regulated by the specific HIV DNA polymerase: reverse transcriptase. If a DNA copy is not formed, the viral RNA genome becomes susceptible to destruction by cellular enzymes. The nucleoside reverse transcriptase inhibitors are both competitive inhibitors of reverse transcriptase and DNA chain terminators. The normal $2'$ deoxynucleosides, which are substrates for DNA synthesis, link to form a chain by phosphodiester linkages bridging the $5'$ and $3'$ positions on the five-carbon sugar molecule. The $2',3'$-dideoxynucleoside analogues are formed by the replacement of the $3'$-hydroxy group by an azido (zidovudine), hydrogen or other group. These nucleoside analogues as substrates will bind to the active site of the HIV reverse transcriptase and will be added to the growing HIV proviral DNA chain. However, once inserted, the normal $5'$ to $3'$ links will not occur, resulting in HIV proviral DNA chain termination. Genotypic mutations at various codons in the reverse transcriptase gene result in decreased susceptibility of HIV to inhibition by the nucleoside reverse transcriptase inhibitors. Several nucleoside reverse transcriptase inhibitors are currently licensed (Table 19.1).

The primary mechanism for toxicities of NRTIs is via mitochondrial damage due to the incorporation of NRTIs into mitochondrial DNA by DNA polymerase. This can manifest clinically as peripheral neuropathy, myopathy, pancreatitis, hepatic steatosis and rarely lactic acidosis. Consequently, dideoxynucleosides are no longer recommended treatment options. Newer agents such as tenofovir and abacavir are thought to cause less mitochondrial damage. Thymidine analogues such as D4T and AZT are usually avoided as they have been shown to be the main cause of facial and limb fat loss (lipotrophy).

The use of abacavir should be limited to those who are HLA B*5701 negative as they are significantly less likely to experience a hypersensitivity reaction, which occurs most commonly within the first 6 weeks of therapy. Owing to recently published data, caution should be applied when prescribing abacavir in patients with a high

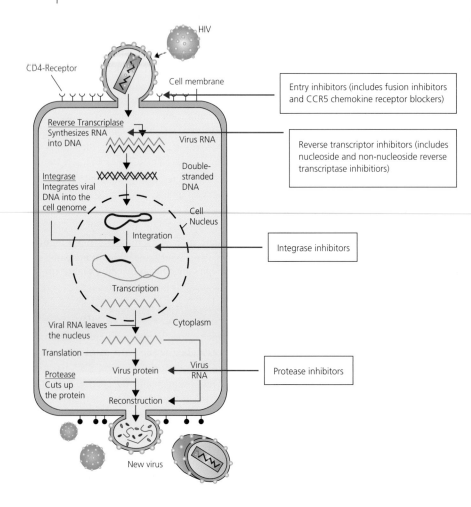

**Figure 19.1** Targets for combination antiretroviral therapy in HIV life cycle.

**Table 19.1** Antiretrovirals licensed for use in UK: 2011.

| Nucleos(t)ides | Non-nucleosides | Protease inhibitors | Integrase inhibitors | Fusion or entry inhibitors |
|---|---|---|---|---|
| Zidovudine | Nevirapine | Amprenavir | Raltegravir | Enfurvitide |
| Lamivudine | Efavirenz | Fosamprenavir | | Maraviroc |
| Abacavir | Etravirine | Atazanavir | | |
| Emtricitabine | Rilpivirine | Darunavir | | |
| Stavudine | Delavirdine | Indinavir | | |
| Didanosine | | Lopinavir and | | |
| Tenofovir | | ritonavir | | |
| | | Nelfinavir | | |
| | | Ritonavir | | |
| | | Saquinavir | | |
| | | Tipranavir | | |

Fixed dose pill formulations: Atripla (tenofovir, emtricitabine, efavirenz); Truvada (tenofovir, emtricitabine); Kivexa (abacavir, lamivudine); Combivir (zidovudine, lamivudine); Kaletra (lopinavir/ritonavir), Eviplera (tenofovir, emtricitabine, efavirenz).

cardiovascular risk and/or patients with a plasma viral load greater than 100 000 copies/mL.

The non-nucleoside reverse transcriptase inhibitors are a group of structurally diverse agents that bind to reverse transcriptase at a site distant to the active site resulting in conformational changes at the active site and inhibition of enzyme activity. These agents show high antiviral activity *in vitro* and have relatively low toxicity. They are also highly specific, inhibiting the reverse transcriptase of HIV-1 but not HIV-2. In monotherapy, rapid emergence of resistant strains associated with single point mutations of the reverse transcriptase gene, high level phenotypic resistance and loss of antiviral effect occur. The drugs therefore need to be combined with other antiretroviral agents, usually two nucleoside/tide reverse transcriptase inhibitors, to achieve and maintain an effective long-term treatment response. Rash and hepatitis can occur with all non-nucleoside therapy. A greater risk of hepatotoxicity has been reported with nevirapine, particularly in patients with higher CD4 counts. Vivid dreams, insomnia and other CNS side effects are well described with efavirenz.

## Protease inhibitors

The protease inhibitors (PIs) bind competitively to the substrate site of the viral protease. This enzyme is responsible for the post-translational processing and cleavage of a large structural core protein during budding from the infected cell. Inhibition results in the production of immature virus particles that are unable to infect other target cells. Pharmacokinetic enhancement of PIs by concomitant administration of low-dose ritonavir permits lower pill burden and a higher genetic barrier to the development of resistance. This is due to the ability of ritonavir to inhibit cytochrome P450-mediated metabolism of PIs. Metabolic complications such as insulin resistance, hyperlipidaemia and truncal fat accumulation (lipohypertrophy/lipodystrophy) are well described with protease inhibitors. Other important complications include an increased cardiovascular risk and nephrolithiasis.

## Integrase inhibitors

The integration of the viral DNA into the host chromosome is achieved through a process of DNA splicing and recombination. First, two nucleotides are removed from each 3′-end of the viral DNA, a process termed 3′-end processing. In the second step, termed DNA strand transfer, the processed viral DNA ends are inserted or joined into the host DNA. The HIV-1 integrase catalyses these first two steps of integration. In the third step, cellular enzymes repair the single gaps in the DNA chain by removing the two unpaired nucleotides at the 5′-ends of the viral DNA. The integrase inhibitors raltegravir and elvitegravir both impede viral replication by inhibiting strand transfer. They are well tolerated and recent studies have confirmed similar efficacy to other first-line regimens with fewer potential drug–drug interactions as they are not metabolized via the cytochrome P450-mediated pathway. These properties have led to their inclusion as first-line therapy in recent guidelines.

## Chemokine receptor antagonists

Chemokine receptors CCR5 and CXCR4 act as co-receptors to facilitate HIV viral entry into host cells. HIV isolates can be divided into R5 and X4 strains depending on which co-receptor they use. The majority of strains utilise CCR5 but X4 using strains may develop in patients who have had a low CD4 count or longer duration of HIV infection. Resistance testing using tropism assays is recommended prior to initiating therapy (see Chapter 3).

## Fusion inhibitors

Enfurvitide (T20) is a fusion inhibitor that prevents entry of HIV into the cell by binding to the viral protein gp41, preventing binding of gp120 to the CD4 receptor. T20 is administered twice daily by subcutaneous injection and its use is currently limited to those with multidrug-resistant HIV. T20's main side effect is local injection site reactions.

## Other treatment modalities

Trials have shown that although treatment with cycles of the cytokine interleukin 2 results in substantial increase in CD4 counts, there is no clinical benefit when used with combination antiretroviral therapy (cART). Therapeutic vaccines have had similar disappointing results. Research is ongoing to develop drugs that can activate latent HIV which, if possible, offer the potential to eradicate HIV infection.

## Treatment of chronic adult infection

In the mid-1990s, several large clinical endpoint studies demonstrated a strong association between falls in plasma HIV RNA levels (plasma viral load) in the first few weeks on therapy and clinical outcome at 1 year. It is now accepted that falls in plasma viral load combined with increases in CD4 count are predictive of the clinical treatment response on different combination regimens at 1–2 years, although changes in the markers probably do not fully predict the observed clinical effect. Where possible an objective of cART is to reduce and sustain plasma viral load levels to below the level of detectability of the current ultrasensitive viral load assays (<50 copies/mL). If patients are adherent to therapy, the likelihood of a viral load rebound and drug resistance is minimal. Despite inhibition of viral replication in plasma, lymph nodes and at other sites, reservoirs of HIV infection in latently infected resting T lymphocytes remain. Continued activation of these cells will theoretically result in the reduction of this reservoir; however, new cells probably continue to be infected as a result of either localized small bursts of viral replication or loss of the antiretroviral effect of the treatment regimen. Even in patients who have sustained, undetectable levels of plasma viral load (<50 copies/mL) for 3 years or more, discontinuation of cART results in rapid rebound of plasma viral load to pre-treatment levels with an increased risk of HIV and non-HIV-related clinical disease. The optimal time to initiate therapy with the current antiretroviral drugs has not been established in clinical studies. CD4 count and plasma viral load are predictors of the estimated risk of progression to AIDS, which is a factor in determining when to start treatment. The motivation of a patient to start and adhere to therapy and the known effectiveness of current regimens are also important.

## When to start therapy (Table 19.2)

Clinical practice across Europe and North America varies, but most clinicians would consider initiating therapy at some point when the CD4 count is less than $500 \times 10^6$/L and in all patients who have symptomatic HIV disease. There is emerging data highlighting benefit of cART during primary HIV infection (PHI). UK guidelines (BHIVA, 2012) recommend initiating cART if PHI is severe (neurological involvement, the presence of an AIDS-defining illness, or a low CD4 count (<350 cells/µL). In addition, it is suggested that cART should be considered if the HIV diagnosis is made very soon after HIV acquisition (<12 weeks).

Treatment of HIV has been shown to reduce HIV transmission. Specific situations where the initiation of cART may be considered for this purpose include PHI and serodiscordant couples.

## Choice of therapy

Preferred first-line therapies cited in guidelines worldwide are varied and dependent on date of publication. Most guidelines recommend that first-line treatment should consist of three antiretroviral agents, which usually consists of two nucleoside/tides and either a non-nucleoside or a protease inhibitor as the third agent. This is often referred to as HAART or cART. Resistance testing is recommended prior to starting due to risk that patients may have acquired, or developed, drug-resistant virus. Co-formulations of drugs commonly used to treat HIV infection have helped to reduce pill burden and improve adherence.

## Antiretroviral regimens

There are various international antiretroviral treatment guidelines, the British HIV Association Guidelines for treatment of

**Table 19.2** When to start: summary.

| | EACS (1) (2011) | BHIVA (2) (2012) | WHO (2010) (3) | IAS (2011) (4) |
|---|---|---|---|---|
| Symptomatic HIV | Start at any CD4 count | Start at any CD4 count | Start at any CD4 count | Start at any CD4 count |
| Asymptomatic HIV infection | CD4 < 350 cells/µL | CD4 < 350 cells/µL | CD4 ≤ 350 cells/µL | CD4 < 500 cells/µL |
| Special situations | Treatment recommended if hepatitis C coinfection, hepatitis B coinfection requiring therapy, HIV-associated nephropathy or other specific organ deficiency, age >50, pregnancy or malignancy Treatment should be considered for viral load (VL) >$10^5$ c/ml or high cardiovascular risk | Hepatitis B coinfection requiring therapy, pregnancy and CD4 % <14. | Hepatitis B coinfection requiring therapy and pregnancy | All persons with HIVAN, hepatitis B and pregnancy |
| Serodiscordant couples | Offer at any CD4 | Offer at any CD4 | | No specific recommendation |

Adapted from:

1. EACS Guidelines 2011 (www.europeanaidsclinicalsociety.org/Guidelines/G1_p17.htm) (last accessed 10 October 2011).
2. British HIV Association HIV treatment guidelines 2012 (www.bhiva.org).
3. WHO (http://whqlibdoc.who.int/publications/2010/9789241599764_eng.pdf) (last accessed 10 October 2011).
4. http://www.aidsinfo.nih.gov/guidelines/html/1/adult-and-adolescent-treatment-guidelines/29/preventing-secondary-transmission-of-hiv.

**Table 19.3** Initial combination regimen for antiretroviral-naïve patients.

| Select NRTI backbone and either a boosted protease inhibitor, NNRTI or an integrase inhibitor | Preferred | Alternative |
|---|---|---|
| NRTI backbone | Tenofovir & emtricitabine | Abacavir & lamivudine |
| 3rd Agent | Atazanavir/ritonavir Darunavir/ritonavir Efavirenz Raltegravir | Lopinavir/ritonavir Nevirapine Rilpivirine Fosamprenavir/ritonavir |

HIV-infected adults are among the most recent at the time of publication are summarized in Table 19.3.

## Further reading

BHIVA. Treatment Guidelines 2012. (www.bhiva.org).

EACS HIV online treatment guidelines. (www.europeanaidsclinicalsociety.org/Guidelines/index.htm).

Priority interventions HIV/AIDS prevention, treatment and care in the health sector (2010 version). (www.who.int/hiv/pub/guidelines/9789241500234/en/index.html).

http://www.aidsinfo.nih.gov/guidelines/html/1/adult-and-adolescent-treatment-guidelines/29/preventing-secondary-transmission-of-hiv.

# CHAPTER 20

# Pharmacopoeia of Treatments

*J. Minton[1], G. Sethi[2] and S. G. Edwards[3]*

[1]University College London Hospitals NHS Foundation Trust, Mortimer Market Centre, London, UK
[2]Guy's and St Thomas' Hospital, London, UK
[3]Camden Provider Services, Mortimer Market Centre, London, UK

---

## OVERVIEW

- UK and US guidelines support early initiation of cART for most OIs

- The benefits, and timing, of initiation of combination antiretroviral therapy (cART) is not well defined for all opportunistic infections

- Following initiation of successful cART, immune reconstruction can lead to a flare in the severity of the condition being treated. This is known as IRIS (immune reconstitution inflammatory syndrome)

- Many HIV and opportunistic infection therapies are either inhibitors, inducers or substrates of the cytochrome P450 system. Knowledge of drug–drug interaction and common side effects is important to avoid drug prescribing errors and manage drug toxicities

---

This chapter lists disease-specific recommendations for the treatment of the most common opportunistic infections (Table 20.1). Table 20.2 highlights important adverse events and complications of specific drug therapy. Table 20.3 lists renal dosing recommendations for drugs commonly used to treat opportunistic infections (OIs).

## The role of cART after diagnosis of an opportunistic infection

The benefits, and timing, of initiation of cART in the setting of an opportunistic infection is not clearly defined though there is accumulating evidence that prompt initiation of cART reduces mortality in some OIs. In view of this, UK and US guidelines support early initiation of cART in most OIs. Although cART has a clear beneficial role in the treatment of certain opportunistic infections (e.g. cryptosporidiosis, Kaposi sarcoma), the risks and benefits are more finely balanced in other OIs (e.g. cryptococcal meningitis) and can vary depending on the site and severity of the OIs.

Initiating cART leads to an improvement in the immune system which helps to reduce the risk of developing a second OI. However, the resulting immune reconstitution can lead to a flare in the severity of the condition being treated. This is known as IRIS (immune reconstitution inflammatory syndrome). Further problems encountered are drug–drug interactions, overlapping drug toxicity and increased tablet burden, with the concern that this may negatively impact on treatment adherence.

The safety of treatment of opportunistic infections during pregnancy is variable. Many drugs have not had their safety studied in human pregnancy, and there is inadequate data to suggest they are safe to use. In each situation the risks and benefits to both the mother and the baby should be considered. In general, though, the following drugs should be avoided: folate antagonists, ganciclovir, cidofovir, tetracyclines. Up-to-date information on individual drugs should be consulted and is available on www.emc.medicines.org.uk.

---

*ABC of HIV and AIDS*, Sixth Edition. Edited by Michael W. Adler,
Simon G. Edwards, Robert F. Miller, Gulshan Sethi and Ian G. Williams.
© 2012 Blackwell Publishing Ltd. Published 2012 by Blackwell Publishing Ltd.

**Table 20.1** Treatment of opportunistic infections.

| Disease | Treatment | Special considerations |
|---|---|---|
| Pneumocystis pneumonia (PCP) | 1 Co-trimoxazole 120 mg/kg/day po/iv in 2–4 divided doses for 3 days then reduce to 90 mg/kg/day for further 18 days.<br>2 Clindamycin 600 mg QDS or 900 mg TDS IV po/iv + primaquine 15 mg od po for 21 days<br><br>**Alternatives**<br>Pentamidine 4 mg/kg iv od<br>Trimethoprim 20 mg/kg/day po + Dapsone 100 mg od po*<br>Atovaquone 750 mg po bd*<br>(*mild to moderate disease only)<br>Duration of treatment 21 days | Steroids given early in the course of therapy, in addition to PCP treatment have been shown to reduce mortality in cases of moderate to severe disease. They should be given if the patient has: $pO_2$ <9.3 kPa on admission and/or arterial–alveolar oxygen gradient >4.7 kPa.<br>Options include:<br><br>• methylprednisolone 1 g/day iv for 3 days, followed by 0.5 g iv for 2 days, followed by oral prednisolone 80 mg tailing off over 16 days<br>• oral prednisolone 40 mg bd for 5 days then 40 mg daily on days 6–10 and 20 mg daily on days 11–21 |
| | **Prophylaxis**<br>Cotrimoxazole 480 or 960 mg od or 960 mg 3× a week<br>Dapsone 50–100 mg od (+25 mg of pyrimethamine 3× a week if positive toxoplasmosis serology)<br>Nebulized pentamidine 300 mg every 2–4 weeks<br>Atovoquone: 750 mg bd | Indications for starting primary prophylaxis include:<br><br>• CD4 <200 cells/µL or CD4% <14%<br>• persistent oral candida<br>• AIDS-defining illness<br><br>Caution starting cART regimens and co-trimoxazole concomitantly as, if rash occurs, it creates confusion as to cause and may limit future antiretroviral options<br>Discontinue secondary prophylaxis for patients on cART with increase in CD4 count >200 cells/µL AND undetectable plasma HIV RNA for at least 3 months |
| Toxoplasmosis | 1 Sulfadiazine 6 g/day in 2–4 divided doses po for 6 weeks<br>2 Clindamycin 600 mg qds iv/po<br><br>Above are given with Pyrimethamine (200-mg loading dose followed by 50 mg od po) + folinic acid 15 mg/day po<br>Alternative, less-studied regimens include clarithromycin + minocycline, and atovoquone + minocycline<br><br>**Prophylaxis:**<br>Sulfadiazine 500 mg qds po or clindamycin 300 mg qds with Pyrimethamine 25 mg od + folinic acid 10–15 mg/day | Consideration should be given to weight-based dosing of sulfadiazine 15 mg/kg qds (max. dose 100 mg/kg/day)<br>Cerebral toxoplasmosis:<br><br>• brain imaging is required at 2–3 weeks to assess response to treatment. Consider brain biopsy if lack of response at 3 weeks or clinical deterioration.<br>• Use of steroids may complicate assessment of clinical response and should be avoided if possible.<br>• Longer courses of treatment may be considered for slow response.<br><br>Discontinue secondary prophylaxis for patients on cART with increase in CD4 count >200 cells/µL AND undetectable plasma HIV RNA for at least 3–6 months<br>Anticonvulsant therapy may be needed for seizure control. Sodium Valproate or Levetiracetam are preferred as they have fewer interactions with cART<br>Folinic acid is given prophylactically to reduce the potential for pyrimethamine induced myelosuppression. DO NOT GIVE FOLIC ACID |
| Cytomegalovirus | Treatment<br>Ganciclovir 5 mg/kg iv bd<br>or<br>Valganciclovir 900 mg po bd<br>or<br>Foscarnet 90 mg/kg iv bd<br>or<br>Cidofovir 5 mg/kg/week iv for 2 doses and then reduce to fortnightly<br><br>**Prophylaxis**<br>Ganciclovir 5 mg/kg iv od<br>Valganciclovir 450 mg bd<br>Foscarnet 90 mg/kg iv od<br>Cidofovir 5 mg/kg iv fortnightly | Correct dosing and administration of all agents complex. See www.emc.medicines.org.uk and/or seek advice of HIV specialist pharmacist prior to prescribing. Adjust dose of all agents according to renal function.<br><br>Give probenecid 2 g and iv hydration prior to cidofovir<br>Treatment should be continued for 21 days.<br><br>**CMV retinitis**<br>Prophylaxis required to reduce the risk of recurrence. Following advice from ophthalmologist prophylaxis may be discontinued for patients on cART with increase in CD4 count >100 cells/µL AND undetectable plasma HIV RNA for at least 3 months |

**Table 20.1** *(continued)*

| Disease | Treatment | | Special considerations |
|---------|-----------|---|------------------------|
| Cryptococcus | In severe disease:<br>Liposomal amphoteracin B 4 mg/kg/day iv plus flucytosine 25 mg/kg qid iv ×2 weeks followed by fluconazole 400–800 mg/day po for an additional 8 weeks<br>Fluconazole 400 mg/day alone may be used for less severe disease<br>Prophylaxis<br>Fluconazole 200-400 mg daily po | | Amphotericin B 0.7–1.0 mg/kg qd iv may be used if access to liposomal formulation not available<br>If cerebrospinal fluid (CSF) pressure raised consider daily lumbar puncture or CSF shunt<br>Serum CrAg not helpful in monitoring response to treatment or identification or relapse |
| Candida | Fluconazole 50–100 mg/day po (up to maximum of 400 mg daily)<br>Itraconazole solution 100–200 mg bd po<br>If no clinical response test for resistance and consider:<br>Amphotericin iv<br>Voriconazole<br>Caspofungin | | There may be complex interactions between antifungals and cART see www.emc.medicines.org.uk/for more information |
| Cryptosporidiosis | cART | | Improvement of the immune system is the most effective therapy |
| Herpes simplex virus encephalitis | Aciclovir 10 mg/kg iv three times a day for 7–10 days | | Consider Foscarnet 120–180 mg/kg/day iv in 2 or 3 daily doses for treatment failure (see above for advice on renal dosing) |
| *Mycobacterium tuberculosis* | Rifampicin<br><br>Isoniazid +<br>Pyridoxine<br>Pyrazinamide<br><br>Ethambutol | 600 mg po daily if patient ≥50 kg<br>450 mg po daily if patient <50 kg<br>300 mg po daily<br>10–25 mg po daily<br>2 g po daily if patient ≥50 kg<br>1.5 g po daily if patient <50 kg<br>15 mg/kg po daily | Quadruple therapy used as initial therapy in HIV related TB – as in the general population<br>Patients should be counselled about possible visual changes that can occur with ethambutol<br>Explain that bodily secretions will be discoloured red with rifampicin and that soft contact lenses may be permanently stained<br>Advise that barrier methods of contraception will be needed if using hormonal contraception (and for up to 4 weeks after stopping rifampicin)<br>Directly observed therapy (DOT) should be considered for selected patients<br>Complex interactions between rifamycin and cART. |
| *Mycobacterium avium* | Ethambutol 15 mg/kg po daily<br>Clarithromycin 500 mg po once or twice daily<br>Rifabutin 300 mg po daily*<br>Amikacin 7.5 mg/kg/day iv as a single dose for 28 days*<br>*Consider if disease severe or refractory to oral treatment | | Uveitis risk increases with rifabutin and clarithromycin<br>Complex interactions between rifamycin and all cART regimens |
| Microsporidia | cART | | Improvement of the immune system is the most effective therapy |
| Aspergillosis | Voriconazole 6 mg/kg every 12 hours (for the first 24 hours) then 4 mg/kg twice a day for at least 7 days, followed by 200 mg orally twice a day to complete a total of 12 weeks therapy<br><br>**Alternatives**<br>Liposomal amphotericin 3 mg/kg/day<br>Caspofungin 70 mg on day 1 followed by 50 mg od (70 mg if >80 kg)<br>Treatment regimens above usually given until treatment response and then followed by itraconazole solution 200 mg bd po or voriconazole 200 mg bd po for up to 12 weeks | | Initial treatment intravenous, followed by oral therapy<br>Caspofungin, Voriconazole and Itraconazole have interactions with cART regimens |
| Histoplasmosis | Liposomal amphotericin 3 mg/kg/day followed by itraconazole solution 200 mg bd<br>Minimum 12 weeks therapy. Consider long-term itraconazole | | Consider itraconazole levels<br>cART |

**Table 20.2** Principle adverse events of drugs commonly used in the treatment of opportunistic infections. More detailed information is available on www.emc.medicines.org.uk.

| Drug | Adverse events | Precautions for use |
| --- | --- | --- |
| Co-trimoxazole | Nausea and vomiting, leucopenia and rash (rarely Stevens–Johnson syndrome and toxic epidermal necrolysis) Hepatitis, thrombocytopenia, hyperkalaemia | Avoid (or extreme caution) in patients with G6PD deficiency Reduce dose in renal impairment Avoid in severe liver disease zidovudine: ↑ risk myelosuppression |
| Clindamycin | Nausea, vomiting, abdominal discomfort, loose stools, diarrhoea (may cause overgrowth of *Clostridium difficile*), rash and abnormal liver function tests | |
| Primaquine | Nausea, vomiting, methaemoglobinaemia, anaemia, neutropenia, agranulocytosis, cardiac arrhythmias and hypertension | Haemolytic anaemia can occur in G6PD deficiency zidovudine: ↑ risk myelosuppression |
| Dapsone | Nausea, vomiting, anorexia, headache, hepatitis, psychosis, haemolysis and methaemoglobinaemia (generally in patients given more than 200 mg/day), and aplastic anaemia. Rash, pruritus, and serious cutaneous hypersensitivity reactions including Stevens–Johnson syndrome. Peripheral neuropathy with motor loss | Rifampicin: ↓↓ levels dapsone Avoid drugs known to cause peripheral neuropathy Drugs that increase gastric pH lower dapsone absorption |
| Pentamidine iv | Pancreatitis, hyper and hypoglycaemia, electrolyte abnormalities, diabetes, hypotension, acute renal failure, cardiac arrhythmias, flushing, rash, dizziness, hepatitis | Pre-hydrate with normal saline to ↓ risk nephrotoxicity Regular monitoring of full blood count, electrolytes, glucose, calcium, magnesium and liver function Avoid nephrotoxic drugs |
| Pentamidine nebulized | Bronchospasm Lower incidence of systemic side effects (see above) | Pentamidine inhalation may provoke cough. Avoid in patients potentially infected with active TB. Procedure should be carried out in a negative flow room and all precautions for minimizing the risk of TB transmission must be followed ↑ risk of PCP in upper lobes of lung Give salbutamol 2.5 mg via conventional nebulizer to prevent bronchospasm |
| Pyrimethamine | Rash, atrophic glossitis, abdominal pain, vomiting, megaloblastic anaemia, neutropenia, thrombocytopenia, pancytopenia, headache, dizziness insomnia | Folic acid inhibits action of pyrimethamine – give folinic acid instead zidovudine: ↑ risk myelosuppression |
| Atovaquone | Rash, nausea, increased appetite and weight gain, headache, sinus arrhythmia, dyspepsia, flatulence, hand tremor, insomnia, hyperbilirubinaemia and somnolence, anaemia, neutropenia, hyponatraemia, hepatitis, elevated creatinine kinase | Take with food Should not be used in patients with: severe PCP, malabsorption conditions or pre-existing diarrhoea or in patients who are nil by mouth or not taking oral nutrition Rifampicin: ↓ levels atovaquone |
| Sulfadiazine | Nausea, vomiting, diarrhoea, cyanosis, headache, depression and mental confusion. Other blood dyscrasias including agranulocytosis, aplastic anaemia, leucopenia, and thrombocytopenia, rash (rarely Stevens–Johnson syndrome), hepatitis, jaundice, hepatic necrosis, renal toxicity, necrotizing angiitis with hypersensitivity, pancreatitis and crystalluria | See co-trimoxazole plus Sulfadiazine is a poorly soluble sulphonamide and at high concentrations will precipitate in urine. It is essential to maintain a good fluid input po/iv with a urine output of at least 3 L per day during treatment |
| Ganciclovir | Neutropenia, thrombocytopenia, anaemia, eosinophilia, fever, rash, abnormal liver function tests (LFTs), raised urea or creatinine | Reduce dose in renal impairment zidovudine: ↑ risk myelosuppression Caution using myelosuppressive and nephrotoxic drugs Because of the mutagenic and teratogenic potential of ganciclovir, women of childbearing potential should be advised to use effective contraception during treatment |
| Cidofovir | Proteinuria, fever, neutropenia, asthenia, nausea with vomiting, rash, nephrotoxicity, dyspnoea, pneumonia, decreased intraocular pressure, nephrogenic diabetes insipidus | Administered in conjunction with oral probenecid and iv hydration Adjust dose in renal impairment Avoid concurrent nephrotoxic drugs |
| Foscarnet | Nephrotoxicity, electrolyte abnormalities headache, nausea and vomiting, fatigue, rash, convulsion, genital ulceration, anaemia | Adjust dose in renal impairment. Avoid concurrent nephrotoxic drugs Foscarnet solution 24 mg/mL is given over 2 hours with 1 L of 0.9% sodium chloride. If it is being given peripherally it is important that the 1 L of 0.9% sodium chloride runs concurrently with the foscarnet to reduce the incidence of thrombophlebitis |

**Table 20.2** (continued)

| Drug | Adverse events | Precautions for use |
|---|---|---|
| Fluconazole | Gastrointestinal side effects more common at doses >600 mg od and include nausea, abdominal discomfort, diarrhoea and flatulence, dry mouth, raised liver enzymes, haematological side effects | |
| Voriconazole | See fluconazole plus visual disturbances including altered perception, blurred vision, changes in coloured vision and photophobia (usually transient and reversible) | Complex drug interactions with antiretrovirals see www.emc.medicines.org.uk/ |
| Caspofungin | Nausea, vomiting, abdominal pain, diarrhoea, flushing, fever, headache, injection site reactions, rash, pruritus, anaemia; also reported, pulmonary oedema, adult respiratory distress syndrome, hypersensitivity reactions (including anaphylaxis) | Administer iv in 250 mL of sodium chloride 0.9% (incompatible with glucose solutions) Has no activity against cryptococcus |
| Amphoteracin | Fever (sometimes with shaking chills), headache, anorexia, nausea and vomiting, malaise, muscle and joint pain, venous pain at the injection site with phlebitis, and thrombophlebitis. Abnormal renal function, hypokalaemia and hypomagnesaemia, acute liver failure, normochromic normocytic anaemia, thrombocytopenia, leucopenia and other haematological toxicities | A test dose of amphotericin 1 mg infused over 20–30 min should be given before commencing treatment Incompatible with sodium chloride 0.9% Lower risk of renal impairment with lipid formulations Adjust dose in renal impairment Avoid myelosuppressive and nephrotoxic drugs There is a theoretical interaction between the modes of action of amphotericin and fluconazole, which contraindicates their use together |
| Rifampicin | Flushing, itching, rash, anorexia, nausea, vomiting, abdominal discomfort, diarrhoea, hepatitis, hyperbilirubinaemia, thrombocytopenia, leucopenia, haemolytic anaemia, eosinophilia, oedema and muscle weakness. Reddish discolouration of urine, sputum and tears. Soft contact lenses may be permanently stained | Rifampicin induces hepatic microsomal enzymes and can therefore accelerate the metabolism of many drugs. Check for drug interactions when prescribing cART. In particular, avoid co-prescribing protease inhibitors |
| Rifabutin | Nausea, vomiting, discolouration of skin and urine (orange), increased LFTs, anaemia, and leucopenia. At high doses polyarthralgia/arthritis, transient aphthous stomatitis and uveitis have been reported | Complex interactions between rifamycin and all cART regimens |
| Isoniazid | Peripheral neuritis, transient increases in liver enzymes, hepatic necrosis, anaemia, agranulocytosis, thrombocytopenia, and eosinophilia. Hypersensitivity reactions including skin eruptions, fever, lymphadenopathy and vasculitis. Other side effects include nausea, vomiting, hyperglycaemia, metabolic acidosis, lupus-like-syndrome, optic neuritis, rheumatoid syndrome, urinary retention, and gynaecomastia | |
| Pyrazinamide | A hepatic reaction is the most common side effect. Other side effects include active gout, sideroblastic anaemia, arthralgias, anorexia, nausea, vomiting, dysuria, malaise, fever, urticaria and aggravation of peptic ulcer | |
| Ethambutol | Blurred vision, decreased visual acuity, central scotomas, loss of the ability to detect green or red, peripheral field defects (usually at higher doses) and numbness and paraesthesia of the extremities | |
| Aciclovir | Renal impairment, increased LFTs, reversible neurological complications, i.e. confusion, hallucinations, agitation, tremors, somnolence, psychosis, convulsions and coma, nausea and vomiting, rashes, fevers and decreases in haematological indices | Adjust dose in renal impairment |
| Liposomal anthracyclines | Nausea, vomiting, myelosuppression, hypotension, hand/foot syndrome | Protease inhibitor based therapy may enhance toxicity |
| Paclitaxel | Allergic reactions, alopecia, myalgia, myelosuppression | Protease inhibitor based therapy may enhance toxicity |

**Table 20.3** Renal dosing recommendations.

| Drug | Renal dosing | |
| --- | --- | --- |
| | **CrCl (ml/min)** | **Dose** |
| Co-trimoxazole | >30 | Standard dose |
| | 15–30 | Half standard dose |
| | <15 | Not recommended |
| Clindamycin | Any | No dose adjustment needed |
| Primaquine | Any | No dose adjustment needed; <1% renal excretion |
| Dapsone | >10 | Standard dose |
| | <10 | 50–100 mg daily. Monitor FBC closely as risk of anaemia is more common. Dapsone and its metabolites are excreted renally, dosage adjustment is needed in patients with renal failure |
| Pentamidine iv | ≥10 | Standard dose |
| | <10 | For life threatening infection: 4 mg/kg/day for 7–10 days then alternate days |
| | | For less severe infection: 4 mg/kg on alternate days |
| Pentamidine nebulized | Any | Standard dose |
| Pyrimethamine | Any | No dose adjustment needed |
| Atovaquone | | Not studied in patients with significant renal impairment. If treatment needed, use with caution and monitor closely |
| Sulfadiazine | | Use with caution in renal impairment as crystalluria may occur |
| Ganciclovir (CMV treatment induction doses) | ≥70 | 5 mg/kg bd |
| | 50–69 | 2.5 mg/kg bd |
| | 25–49 | 2.5 mg/kg od |
| | 10–24 | 1.25 mg/kg od |
| | <10 | 1.25 mg/kg od after haemodialysis |
| Valganciclovir (CMV treatment induction doses) | ≥60 | 900 mg bd |
| | 40–59 | 450 mg bd |
| | 25–39 | 450 mg od |
| | 10–24 | 450 mg every 2 days |
| | <10 | 450 mg 2 or 3 times a week post dialysis has been used. No dose recommendation available |
| Cidofovir | ≤55 mL/min or Cr >133 μmol/L | Not recommended. Consult product literature for more information |
| Foscarnet | Dose in mg/kg adjusted according to CrCl/kg Nor recommended if CrCl/kg <0.4 mL/min/kg | Consult product information for more specific information |
| Fluconazole | >10 | Standard dose |
| | ≤10 (no dialysis) | Half standard dose |
| | Regular dialysis | Standard dose after each dialysis session (3× a week) |
| Voriconazole (oral) | Any | No dose adjustment needed |
| Voriconazole (iv) | <50 | The oral preparation should be used as accumulation of the intravenous vehicle occurs |
| Caspofungin | Any | No dose adjustment needed |
| Amphotericin | | Amphotericin is known to be nephrotoxic. Consult product specific information or guidelines for more specific recommendations |
| Flucytosine | >40 | Standard dose |
| | ≥20–40 | Standard dose every 12 hours |
| | ≥10–20 | Standard dose every 24 hours |
| | <10 | Give initial standard dose and then dose according to levels |
| Rifampicin | ≥10 | Standard dose |
| | <10 | 50–100% dose |
| Rifabutin | ≥30 | Standard dose |
| | <30 | Half standard dose to maximum 300 mg a day (before drug interactions are taken into consideration) |
| Isoniazid | ≥10 | Standard dose |
| | <10 | 200–300 mg daily. Give dose post dialysis |

**Table 20.3** *(continued)*

| Drug | Renal dosing | |
|------|-------------|---|
| | **CrCl (ml/min)** | **Dose** |
| Pyrazinamide | Any<br>Consider dose reduction if <10 | No dose adjustment needed |
| Ethambutol | ≥20<br>10–20<br><10 | Standard dose<br>Standard dose every 24–36 hours or 7.5–15 mg/kg/day<br>Standard dose every 48 hours or 5–7.5 mg/kg/day |
| Aciclovir – intravenous | ≥50<br>25–50<br>10–25<br><10 | Standard dose<br>Standard dose every 12 hours<br>Standard dose every 24 hours<br>CAPD: half dose every 24 hours<br>Haemodialysis: as for CAPD, but give post dialysis on dialysis days |

CrCL, creatinine clearance.
US PHS/CDC 2012 guidelines.

## Further reading and resources

Ashley C, Currie A. *Renal Drug Handbook*, 3rd edn. Radcliffe, 2009.

BHIVA. Guidelines for the Treatment of Opportunistic Infection in HIV-seropositive Individuals, 2011. (http://www.bhiva.org/documents/Guidelines/OI/hiv_v12_is2_Iss2Press_Text.pdf).

Infections Diseases Society of America. IDSA Practice Guidelines (http://www.idsociety.org/IDSA_Practice_Guidelines).

www.emc.medicines.org.uk.

www.hiv-druginteractions.org.

www.tthhivclinic.com.

# CHAPTER 21

# Psychological and Mental Health Issues

*B. Hedge*

St Helens and Knowsley Teaching Hospitals NHS Trust, Merseyside, UK

---

**OVERVIEW**

- HIV is now regarded as a lifelong chronic condition for which combination antiretroviral therapy (cART) can prolong life
- The challenge of living with HIV continues to have a negative psychological impact on those infected, their partners and families
- Although many people living with HIV show great resilience to adversity there remains a high level of psychological morbidity
- Psychological interventions can reduce psychological pathology and increase quality of life
- Best clinical practice provides a comprehensive integrated physical and psychosocial care package throughout all phases of disease

---

**Mental health is a state of well-being in which the individual realizes his or her own abilities, can cope with the normal stresses of life, can work productively and fruitfully and is able to make a contribution to his or her community.**

*Source:* (WHO, 2007)

## Psychological wellbeing

Psychological wellbeing is more than the absence of psychopathology. It is the outcome of high-quality experiences in important aspects of life such as work, social, leisure, relationships, sex and self-determination. In order to achieve wellbeing, individuals require the ability to cope with the stressors that life brings them. Coping can be facilitated by good social support.

## Psychological sequelae

Psychological disturbance in people living with HIV (PLWH) ranges from mild distress to major psychiatric pathology. Elevated rates of anxiety, depression, suicidal thoughts, ideation and activation, and post-traumatic stress are reported at all stages of HIV disease.

---

*ABC of HIV and AIDS*, Sixth Edition. Edited by Michael W. Adler,
Simon G. Edwards, Robert F. Miller, Gulshan Sethi and Ian G. Williams.
© 2012 Blackwell Publishing Ltd. Published 2012 by Blackwell Publishing Ltd.

The severity of psychological symptomatology is related to a person's pre-existing vulnerability, past traumatic experiences, their current life circumstances and to their experience of living with HIV. Psychological symptoms can be directly associated with HIV disease, a complication of physical illness or coincidentally associated with HIV. In all cases, psychological symptoms can cause or exacerbate somatic symptoms such as fatigue, malaise or pain. Specific events, e.g. the diagnosis of HIV and significant declines in health, particularly those requiring the commencement of combination antiretroviral therapy (cART) or changes to medication regimens can be particularly stressful (Box 21.1).

---

Box 21.1 **Challenges faced by PLWH**

In addition to the normal stressors of living, PLWH have to live and cope with:

- managing a chronic medical condition
- uncertainty
- physical symptoms of HIV and the side effects of treatments
- changes to appearance
- adherence to medication regimens
- sex and relationships
- disclosure
- stigma

---

## Adjustment to diagnosis

Even when a positive HIV diagnosis is expected, the confirmation of a positive HIV status frequently brings a reaction of shock. Mood disorders including depressive thoughts and fears and anxieties of what the future might hold are common. Individuals frequently anticipate being rejected if they disclose their positive status. For some, low self-esteem is engendered by feelings of shame and guilt at having becoming infected. Others may experience anger and desire retribution from those they believe infected them.

## Physical health

The overall burden of physical symptoms is associated with psychological distress and reduced quality of life. Additionally, the side effects of medications can have both direct psychological effects, e.g. on mood change, altered dreams, and indirect psychological effects, e.g. through the demands of treatment regimens and the negative appraisal of changes to appearance.

## Treatment regimens

The most effective medications are those that both show efficacy and that a PLWH will take in the prescribed manner. Long-term adherence to cART is required to maintain viral suppression. However, more than 30% of users report non-adherence at some time over a 10-year period. Adherence is frequently unintentional but may be intentional when it brings desired outcomes in the short term. Many factors contribute to a person's ability and motivation to adhere to a medication regimen. Adherence can prove difficult, as regimens may require lifestyle changes, prescriptions to be filled, the need to remember to take pills on a regular basis and medications may have adverse side effects. To ensure long-term adherence, access to clear, accurate information and support is essential. In addition, motivational and practical issues that might impact on continued adherence need to be addressed. Consideration of the impact of a treatment regimen as well as its efficacy before it is recommended for a particular person can be beneficial (Figure 21.1).

## Changes to body shape

Changes to physical appearance are among the most stigmatizing adverse events for PLWH, as they can be perceived as disclosing their HIV status. Some medications result in lipodystrophy, which can include fat loss (lipoatrophy) from parts of the body or fat deposition (lipohypertrophy) in other areas. The resulting changes in fat deposition visibly alter a person's appearance. Increased levels of anxiety and depression are found in those with physical changes to body shape. Self-esteem is decreased and more difficulties with sex and relationships are reported (Figure 21.2).

## HIV-associated neurocognitive disorders

With increased life expectancy the cumulative prevalence of HIV-associated neurocognitive disorders (HAND) has risen; some

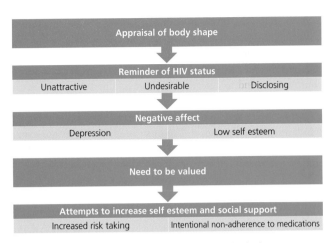

**Figure 21.2** Effects of perceived negative changes to body shape.

studies suggesting that up to 50% of PLWH have some cognitive impairment. There is increasing interest in the early initiation of cART to prevent HAND. The extent to which cognitive deficits can be reversed by later introduction of effective cART is not yet clear (see Chapter 12).

The cognitive deficits seen range from mild to severe and include impairment to attention, memory, learning, language, psychomotor abilities, planning, evaluating, and problem solving; all of which negatively affect wellbeing and independent survival.

## Recognition of psychological symptomatology

Most HIV care is delivered in medical settings. Psychological distress and cognitive deficits are rarely the focus of the visit and frequently go unnoticed. To increase recognition of mental health issues the introduction of routine psychological screening is required on a regular basis. Completion of a comprehensive psychological profile on diagnosis should be followed by regular follow-ups, particularly at times of change, either to the course of the illness or to a person's life. Screening cannot replace a full psychological or cognitive

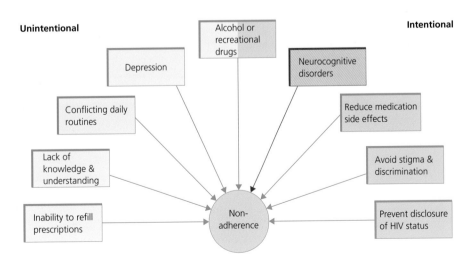

**Figure 21.1** Barriers to adherence.

assessment but can be useful in drawing attention to mental health issues in settings such as GP and HIV clinical consultations.

Open questions concerning the impact of HIV within the context of a person's life, attention to verbal and non-verbal clues during consultations and to changes over time in a person's manner can prove a useful pre-screen.

Formal screening can be conducted through the use of validated standardized questionnaires. These can be administered and scored by a variety of professionals but should be interpreted within the context of a person's life by qualified trained practitioners.

Those with positive screens will require a full psychological assessment in order to elicit the complexities of the distress and co-morbid conditions. Screening can increase the rate of detection of HAND but will need to be followed by a full psychosocial and cognitive assessment in order for the relative impact of emotional and cognitive difficulties within the physical condition and social circumstances to be established (Box 21.2).

---

Box 21.2 **Screening tools**

- Screening tools should be validated for use in those with physical illnesses, and wherever possible for those with HIV. A balance between the resources needed to deliver screening (staff time and training) and the value of information derived from it needs to be established. Suggested brief questionnaires are:

  - Hospital anxiety and depression Scale (HADS)
  - Distress thermometer
  - International HIV Dementia Scale (IHDS)
  - A more detailed screen that is particularly useful for providing a comprehensive baseline of psychological distress and a screen of co-morbid mental health issues is the Client Diagnostic Questionnaire (CDQ).

---

## Psychological Interventions

The main aims of psychological support are to improve mood, decrease stress, increase self-esteem and enhance quality of life, thereby increasing adherence to medication regimens, and reducing risk taking behaviours and the inappropriate use of health-care resources. Psychological support ranges from the provision of information and sign posting to self-help resources, through counselling to impart knowledge, motivate and decrease fears and anxieties, to highly complex structured psychological interventions. Referral to liaison psychiatric services should be available for those with severe psychiatric pathology. Psychological support can usefully be conceptualized as a stepped-care response to a hierarchy of increasing psychological need, required by a decreasing percentage of PLWH.

A variety of individual therapy and group psychological and social support interventions have been shown to be effective in reducing psychological distress and improving adherence to medication regimens (Figure 21.3 and Table 21.1).

## Factors impacting on living with HIV

A number of factors can impact on the experience of living with HIV and the complexities of subsequent psychological management. Some of the most common are:

### Mental illness
Individuals with previously diagnosed mental illness face increased risks of becoming infected with HIV, such as:

- decreased access to HIV prevention materials
- restricted social support

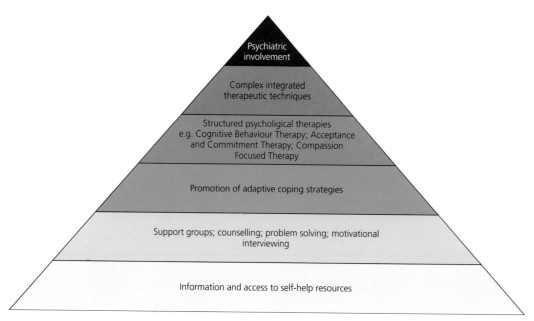

**Figure 21.3** Stepped care model.

**Table 21.1** Psychological interventions.

| Psychological approach | Description | Useful for presentations of |
|---|---|---|
| Psycho-education | Understanding psychological responses to adverse circumstances | Emotional states and unhelpful responses |
| Problem solving and decision making | Consideration of options when none guarantees success | Decisions to be made in the light of uncertainty |
| Anxiety and stress management | Relaxation and breathing strategies | Physiological components of anxiety |
| Behavioural activation | Increasing activity | Depression |
| Cognitive behaviour therapy | Address cognitions; reduce negative emotions; increase adaptive behaviours | Mood disorders; stress and anxiety; non-adaptive coping strategies |
| Acceptance and commitment therapy | Disassociate emotions from negative thoughts | Adjustment to HIV and disease progression |
| Compassion therapy | Stimulates empathy for self; non-judgemental | Living with the negative impact of HIV |
| Systemic approaches | Incorporates interactions between people | Couple, family and caring situations |
| Motivational interviewing | Increases ability for an individual to change unwanted behaviours | Risk behaviours |

- fewer adaptive coping strategies
- co-morbidity with alcohol and substance abuse
- increased incidence of sexual abuse.

Both mental health disorders and substance abuse are found in those diagnosed with HIV. Co-morbidity with mental illness will frequently lead to more complex difficulties in coping with HIV. Living with two stigmatized conditions can adversely affect adherence and clinic attendance, increase risk behaviours and reduce quality of life. There is a need for access to psychological and psychiatric support that is able to address such complex mental health issues within the context of living with HIV.

## Trauma

Previous traumatic life experiences, e.g. violence, torture, sexual assault, natural disasters, particularly when they result in the acquisition of HIV, are associated with an increased incidence of symptoms of post-traumatic stress. Trauma is also associated with an increased incidence of depression, poor adherence and increased risk behaviours. Psychological support that addresses the totality and complexity of a person's experiences is required.

## Individual differences

While HIV presents a number of common challenges to all those infected, individual differences such as ethnicity, gender, sexual orientation, religion and age may pose specific difficulties. Although the majority of those infected with HIV in the UK are men having sex with men, there are increasing numbers of children, older adults, heterosexuals, asylum seekers and refugees whose specific circumstances exacerbate the challenge of living with HIV. Now that women with HIV are living longer, the gender-specific impact of HIV and cART on their immune systems, reproductive systems, cultural and domestic roles and responsibilities is increasingly being realized. It is important that the combined impact of biological, social and psychological factors is recognized and psychological interventions are tailored to meet the needs of individuals within the context of their lives (Figure 21.4).

## Family issues

The psychological needs of both adults and of children living with HIV have separately been well documented. In reality, these needs frequently need to be met simultaneously within a family context. It can be useful for systemic issues to be considered to ensure that practical and psychological support addresses the needs of the whole family.

The implications of being infected with HIV can be extremely distressing for PLWH who are considering having a child, or parenting existing children. Whether children are HIV positive or negative, issues of secrecy, disclosure, illness and mortality may be encountered. When children are HIV positive, the additional difficulties of preparing them for adult life with a chronic disease including acceptance of the responsibility attached to having a transmissible infection have to be addressed. If these issues arise at the same time that young people are transferring from child to adult services, such emotive concerns can easily be overlooked. Wherever possible, young people should have access to multidisciplinary, transitional services that ensure the continuity of clinical and psychological care (Box 21.3).

## Prevention

It remains important that those uninfected by HIV continue to protect themselves from acquiring the virus. However, a multidisciplinary clinic setting provides a timely opportunity to assess sexual and drug using risk behaviours and to offer motivational support for risk reduction with PLWH.

Individuals presenting for post-exposure prophylaxis following sexual exposure (PEPSE) may be in a state of acute anxiety following a failure to maintain safer sexual behaviours. In addition to anxiety management, motivational support, communication and skills enhancement can be offered to reduce the likelihood of further risky sexual behaviours. For those intentionally using PEPSE as an alternative to safer sexual behaviours, information regarding all risks of unsafe sexual behaviours can be given and interventions to motivate the adoption of safer sexual practices can be implemented (Figure 21.5).

| Biological | Social | Psychological | Impact |
|---|---|---|---|
| Direct effects of HIV on women | Roles and responsibilities | Depression exacerbated by HIV diagnosis | Needs relate to health, social and psychological well being |
| Sex specific immune response to cART | Life incompatible with cART regimens | Strees related to social and cultural circumstances | Late presentation |
| Age related hormonal changes | Restricted access to HIV services | Guilt related to the potential to infect child | Non-gender specific clinical care |
| Reproductive issues | Negative power imbalance | Shame of HIV | Dilemmas over decisions related to living with HIV |
| | Socio-cultural norms and expectations | Loss of planned life | Prioritisation of other family members for healthcare |
| | | Grief for lost people, lifestyle and opportunities | Lack of social support |
| | | Fears and anxieties related to stigma, disclosure and future of family | Decrease in quality of life |

**Figure 21.4** Gender inequalities: the impact of HIV on women.

Box 21.3 **Challenges for adolescents with HIV**

Adolescence is the time of:

- transfer of responsibility from a parent to a child
- reduction in parental supervision
- increased opportunities for the child to make decisions
- HIV differentiates from peers
  - denial
  - anger
  - depression
- fear of disclosure of status
  - limited control over environment
  - limited privacy
  - enforced time schedules e.g. school
  - identifiable pill containers
- undesirable side effects from medications
- first sexual relationships
  - coping with safer sex
  - fears of disclosing HIV status
- attempts to gain control
- non-adherence to medication regimens

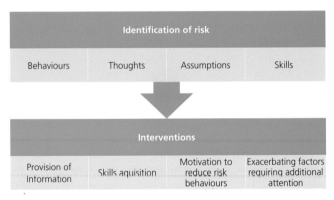

**Figure 21.5** Risk reduction.

will also be infected with HIV. Psychological support for carers is as important as practical support. To ensure that the challenges of living with HIV are seen from the perspective of PLWH it is important that they should be involved in all aspects of service planning. Best clinical practice will be that which integrates the physical and psychological care of PLWH.

Services need to be reactive to the altered psychological needs of PLWH as advances are made in the medical interventions for the treatment and prevention of HIV.

## Service implications

All PLWH require access to regular psychological screening, assessments and a range of psychological support. The burden of care for PLWH frequently falls on partners and families, some of whom

## Further reading

British Psychological Society, British HIV Association & Medical Foundation for AIDS & Sexual Health. *Standards for psychological support for adults living with HIV*. London: MedFASH, 2011.

Catalan J, Meadows J, Douzenis A. The changing patterns of mental health problems in HIV infection: the view from London, UK. *AIDS Care* 2000; 12:222–341.

Johnson WD, Diaz RM, Flanders WD, *et al*. Behavioural interventions to reduce risk for sexual transmission of HIV among men who have sex with men. *Cochrane Database of Systematic Reviews* 2008;3: CD001230.

Lesserman J. Role of depression, stress and trauma in HIV disease progression. *Psychosomatic Med* 2008;70:539–545.

National Institute for Health and Clinical Excellence. *One to one interventions to reduce the transmission of sexually transmitted infections (STIs) including HIV, and to reduce the rate of under 18 conceptions, especially among vulnerable and at risk groups*. NICE public health intervention guidance 3. London: NICE, 2007.

Siegel K, Lekas H. AIDS as a chronic illness: psychosocial implications. *AIDS* 2002;16: S69–S76.

Smart T. *Mental Health and HIV: a critical review. HIV and AIDS*. Treatment in Practice:145. London: NAM, 2009.

WHO. *Mental Health: Strengthening Mental Health Promotion*. Geneva: WHO, 2007.

# CHAPTER 22

# Strategies for Preventing HIV Transmission

*J. Imrie[1,2] and G. J. Hart[1]*

[1] Centre for Sexual Health and HIV Research, University College London, London, UK
[2] Africa Centre for Health and Population Studies, University of KwaZulu-Natal, Somkhele, South Africa

## OVERVIEW

- Sexual health promotion education, promoting condom use, and providing clean needles and syringes are the cornerstones of effective population-level HIV prevention
- Strategies that reduce injecting risk for HIV will have spin-off benefits for reducing other viral infections, for example, hepatitis B and C
- HIV-affected communities, understandably concerned about stigmatization, discrimination and, increasingly, criminalization, can also be prevention's strongest allies when properly engaged
- Effective prevention strategies require combined intervention approaches and clinical sexual health and drug services that are culturally appropriate and show understanding of local epidemiology and context
- Behavioural interventions can be delivered in different settings but must be carefully reviewed before replication in different settings is undertaken
- Risk compensation – increased risky practice sparked by decreased perceived risk – needs to be taken seriously when planning and evaluating prevention programmes

## Introduction

Effective HIV prevention combines health promotion activities that support sustained behaviour change, with biomedical and treatment interventions and high-quality clinical sexual health and drug services. It involves primary and secondary prevention strategies working together. Primary prevention strategies focus on reducing an uninfected person's likelihood of HIV acquisition, while secondary prevention focuses on limiting HIV transmission from those who have the virus. High levels of diagnosed HIV infection, based on high levels of HIV testing, are essential to effective implementation of secondary prevention. Primary and secondary prevention strategies need to be culturally appropriate, age, gender and sexuality specific. They must display understanding of the local epidemiology and the socioeconomic and cultural context where they are to be delivered.

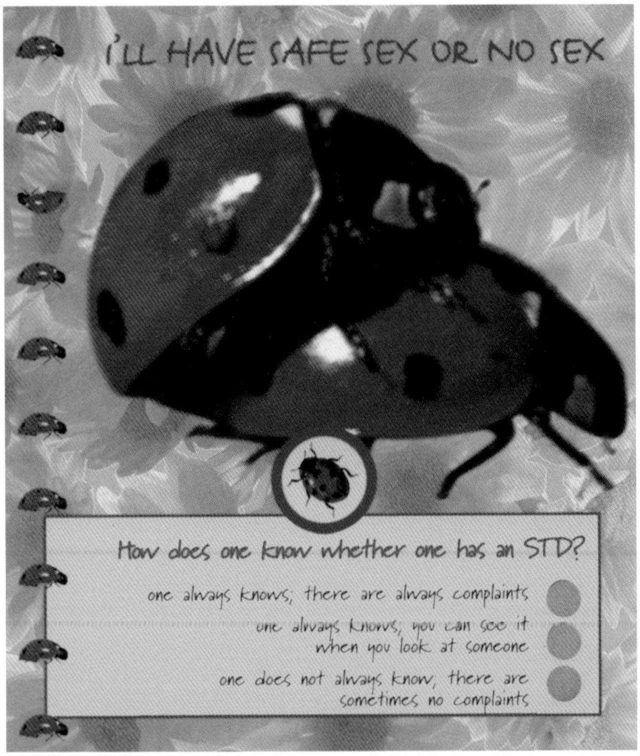

*ABC of HIV and AIDS*, Sixth Edition. Edited by Michael W. Adler,
Simon G. Edwards, Robert F. Miller, Gulshan Sethi and Ian G. Williams.
© 2012 Blackwell Publishing Ltd. Published 2012 by Blackwell Publishing Ltd.

**Figure 22.1** Health education needs to use varied approaches. A Dutch scratch card or following a link to an internet-based quiz (www.avert.org/sexquiz.htm) shows how prevention messages can be delivered in different settings using a range of age appropriate techniques. Reproduced with permission of the Dutch Foundation for STD Control.

This chapter is concerned with prevention in high-income and some middle-income countries, with mature HIV epidemics that are largely concentrated in identifiable subpopulations. However, some principles may be adapted to situations with generalized or still-emerging epidemics. The chapter is concerned exclusively with sexual and parenteral HIV transmission (Figure 22.1).

## Targeted HIV education

HIV education strategies are the cornerstone of focused prevention. Among sexually active people in industrialized countries, knowledge of basic HIV risk reduction strategies, such as consistent condom use, is generally good. But knowledge and practice are rarely well correlated, and safer sex is not consistently practised. The result has been a major increase in rates of sexually transmitted infections (STIs) and unplanned pregnancies. Since the mid-2000s, HIV diagnoses have continued to increase in most industrialized countries largely due to increased numbers presenting for HIV testing; since then, a number of countries have seen small, but sustained reductions in the total number of new diagnoses recorded each year. Despite these variations HIV has remained concentrated in vulnerable minority and subpopulations. It is therefore of limited added benefit to target HIV education at the general population. Resources should instead be used to reach those at greatest risk, usually men who have sex with men (MSM), youth (under 25 years of age), particularly from minority ethnic backgrounds, injecting drug users and, in Europe, black Africans and asylum seekers.

HIV and sexual health education messages need to provide clear information and instruction if promoting behaviour change. Messages that promote condom use or voluntary counselling and testing (VCT) need to give clear directions where to access these services confidentially. Education messages should be delivered in different settings, use a variety of media vehicles, for example school sex education programmes, community outreach organizations and popular television. Messages targeting youth need to sit alongside broader school sex education and start before young people become sexual active. Efficacy of health education relies on it being sustained so individuals move seamlessly from school-based sex education to other community and/or clinic-based programmes that meet their changing needs over the early years of their sexual careers. For this to happen requires political support at all levels, appropriate funding and routine evaluation to ensure programmes meet the changing needs of successive generations (Box 22.1).

---

Box 22.1 **Approaches to sex education most likely to improve sexual health outcomes in young people:**

- Begin early (i.e. sex education should start with pre-teens)
- Cover issues in an incremental and age-appropriate fashion
- Address knowledge and attitudes, and develop participants' practical skills (for example, using condoms)
- Provide information, improve knowledge and build participants' confidence to access sexual health and contraceptive services
- Employ participative approaches extensively (for example, role play)
- Ensure content and delivery are gender sensitive, taking into account the different needs of boys and girls
- Ensure understanding of different sexual choices (for example, delaying first intercourse, resisting pressure for sex) and different sexualities
- Discuss differences in disease burden, for example among minority young people, and foster esteem and social/community awareness
- Deliver interventions in different settings across the community (for example, involve parents and youth services)

---

## Sexual transmission

In industrialized countries, most people diagnosed with HIV infection have acquired it through sexual contact. Populations at greatest risk of sexually transmitted HIV include MSM, sexual partners of injecting drug users and those with history of sexual contacts-from/in Africa. Consistent condom use by commercial sex workers has helped maintain low HIV prevalence in this group, but these are less likely to hold among sex workers in resource-poor settings (Box 22.2).

---

Box 22.2 **Practices that reduce risk for HIV acquisition and transmission**

- Using condoms for all penetrative sexual intercourse
- Reducing numbers of sexual partners
- Using adequate quantities of water-based lubricant for both vaginal and anal intercourse. (Oil-based products will cause latex condoms to perish. Some lubricants containing spermicides can cause irritation and are not recommended for reducing HIV transmission
- Adopting sexual practises that carry a lower risk for HIV transmission (for example, mutual masturbation)
- Avoiding recreational drug use during sexual activity, or when sex is likely to happen
- Ensure timely and routine screening and treatment for other sexually transmitted infections
- For young people, delaying age at which first sexual intercourse takes place is a most effective strategy

---

## Behavioural Interventions

Despite massive expenditure on HIV prevention there is still limited evidence about 'what works' to influence health outcomes at the population level. Evaluation evidence supports the use of targeted interventions, tailored to the cultural context and needs of vulnerable groups. In randomized trials, interventions have been shown to reduce the frequency of sexual risk practices, for example unprotected vaginal or anal intercourse and, in some cases, the incidence of STIs. However, so far none has demonstrated an impact on incidence of HIV infection in an industrialized country context.

Behavioural interventions providing basic HIV prevention skills that include instructions on correct and appropriate condom use enhance motivation for behaviour change, and teach risk reduction and safer sex negotiation skills (including resisting pressure for sex), have had greatest success. Individual interventions may be delivered effectively in different settings – community, small group and one to one. Interventions that are effective in research trials, using proxy measures of HIV transmission risk, may not perform the same in 'real life'. Careful consideration of local epidemiology and a critical assessment of an intervention's generalizability need to precede any resource commitment to a programme that may show little benefit, or worse, a negative impact (Figures 22.2–22.4). The literature contains examples of both (Box 22.3).

## Biomedical and treatment interventions

There is considerable optimism about the potential prevention contribution of biomedical and treatment-based interventions. Recently, both vaginal microbicides and taking anti-HIV therapy in the form of pre-exposure prophylaxis have been shown to be

Box 22.3 **Guidance for enhancing sexual health promotion and HIV prevention in minority ethnic communities**

- Facilitating access to confidential adolescent and adult sexual health and HIV prevention services, making appropriate use of point of care diagnostic tests, and providing services outside routine clinic settings according to the expressed needs of target communities
- Developing materials using language and images appropriate for diverse groups, including non-native English-speakers
- Early and continued sex education in schools to supplement and support provision in the home
- Assisting parents form cultures where sex in general is rarely discussed to discuss sex education
- Providing focused interventions for younger boys in either school or community settings
- Explaining the wider benefits of safer sex in relation to contraception and avoidance of other infections may increase the overall acceptability of messages with all audiences
- Focused work exploring assumptions made about "safe" partners and concurrent relationships where they are common
- Use of appropriate and community-specific delivery points, for example, settings appropriate to the specific culture
- Awareness of different migration, refugee and acculturation experiences between communities and between generations

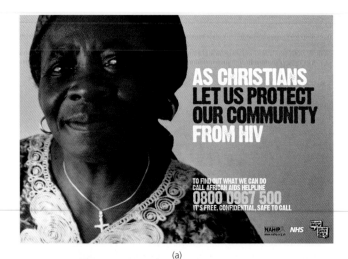

(a)

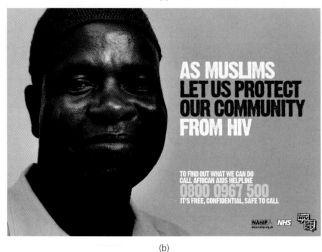

(b)

**Figure 22.3** (a,b) Strategies must demonstrate cultural sensitivity and understanding of context. Campaigns displaying culturally sensitivity are more likely to be perceived as attractive, relevant and meaningful. Reproduced with permission of the National African HIV Prevention Programme, UK.

efficacious in reducing HIV acquisition in certain high-risk populations. However, significant questions about effectiveness at the population level remain, particularly as none of these on their own is likely to be as effective as consistent condom use. Of those available now, only male circumcision, which reduces female-to-male HIV transmission, offers a 'single-shot' prevention intervention. The only partial efficacy of many of the other biomedical interventions means condom use is still required to obtain maximum protective benefit. All biomedical and treatment interventions require initiation of new behaviours that must be sustained. So far biomedical and treatment interventions are not substitutes for

behaviour change and condom use, rather they are additional supplements to mainstream prevention activity.

## Risk compensation

Roll out of behavioural or biomedical prevention strategies needs to proceed cautiously, mindful of the possibility of risk compensation – increases in risky practice sparked by decreases in individuals' perceived risk. The impact of risk compensation has been demonstrated in respect to implementation of seatbelt legislation and failure to reduce road traffic deaths. Although not so well evidenced, there are equally strong arguments about risk compensation in relation to HIV prevention as well.

## Inclusion of people with HIV

HIV-positive people's contribution to HIV prevention has not been adequately recognized. Affected communities are understandably concerned about stigmatization, discrimination and, increasingly,

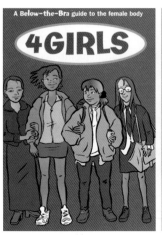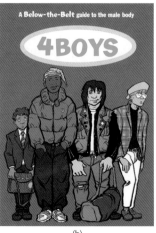

(a)                    (b)

**Figure 22.2** (a,b) Strategies need to be age and gender specific. Sex education content and delivery should be gender sensitive and take account of the different needs of boys and girls. Reproduced with permission from the Family Planning Association.

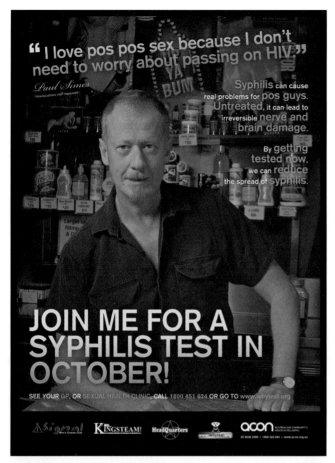

**Figure 22.4** Prevention messages need to offer clear calls to action that are easily enacted 'sex-positive' messages and recognizing the overall importance of sexual health are key in some populations, for example gay and other men who have sex with men. *Source:* Reproduced with permission of ACON – AIDS Council of New South Wales.

criminalization. But properly equipped, they are prevention's strongest allies. Effective positive prevention includes counselling and support in one-to-one and small-group contexts and specialist

sexual health/STI screening services that in addition provide social, emotional and sexual counselling within HIV outpatient treatment services. Interventions to reduce transmission risk, particularly of resistant or virulent HIV strains, are important. These can only happen by engaging people living with HIV. Genuinely productive partnerships with HIV-positive communities are equally essential to overcome social prejudice and stigma issues (Figure 22.4).

## High-quality sexual health services

STIs increase susceptibility of uninfected individuals to HIV and increase the infectiousness of those with HIV. STI control is therefore important in any comprehensive prevention strategy. Clinical services need to provide screening, treatment and partner notification for STIs, as well as high-quality VCT for HIV. Developments in point-of-care HIV testing mean quality services do not need to be limited by available clinic infrastructure, but can be delivered efficiently in different settings, including primary care, tertiary education and community venues. STI screening and treatment offers opportunities for delivering focused behavioural interventions and should be part of routine HIV outpatient treatment services along side appropriate counselling on risk reduction.

## HIV testing

Diagnosis of HIV-infected individuals is most important for secondary prevention. Testing *per se* has only ever been shown to benefit those who test positive – allowing them to benefit from early treatment. Those who test positive are more likely to change their behaviour as a result of their diagnosis. However, there is no comprehensive evidence to indicate that any behaviour change of those who test HIV negative is sustained over time (Figure 22.5). Indeed, there is growing concern that the reverse may apply – those who test negative are more likely to continue to take risks. Brief client-centred counselling as part of routine STI care has been shown to be an

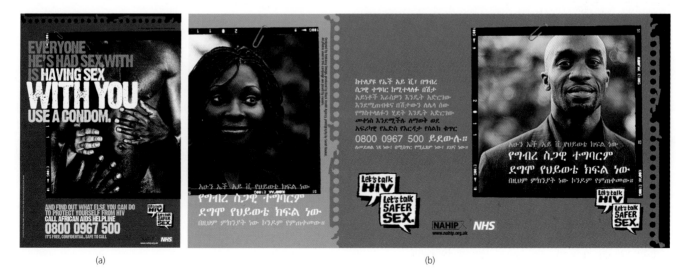

(a)                                    (b)

**Figure 22.5** (a,b) Education campaigns must employ appropriate language and materials, including different formats and languages. *Source:* Reproduced with permission of the National African HIV Prevention Programme, UK.

effective strategy in reducing future STI acquisition in only one trial. Nevertheless, for its benefit to the individual and secondary prevention importance, VCT cannot be ignored and is still an important component of any comprehensive prevention strategy.

## HIV treatment as prevention

There is an accumulating body of evidence that a strategy of early diagnosis and initiation of immediate treatment at a population level may have some success in controlling onward transmission of HIV infection. To improve the chance of success this strategy would need a change in the culture of testing, with increased availability of testing and more people being tested at greater frequency than currently occurs. A willingness of HIV-positive persons to initiate therapy will depend on long-term safety concerns about HIV therapy.

## Parenteral HIV transmission: injecting drug users

HIV transmission between injecting drug users (IDUs) occurs primarily through sharing of contaminated syringes, needles and other injecting equipment. IDUs and their partners are also at risk through sexual transmission, either through commercial sex to support their drug use or from their non-paying partners. The epidemiology of HIV among injecting drug users and the social and cultural context of drug use vary between countries and regions. This must be reflected in local prevention strategies. Promising interventions for a given setting are highly reliant upon understanding local context – epidemiology and drug-use culture (Box 22.4).

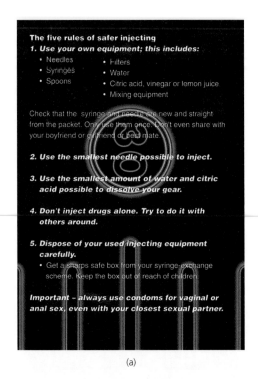

(a)

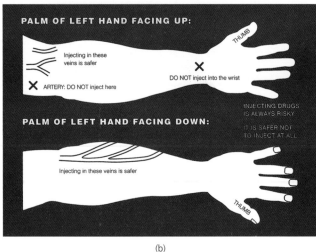

(b)

**Figure 22.6** An example of good practice in provision of effective accurate information for injecting drug users. Reproduced from *A Guide to Safer Injecting* with permission from HIT.

> **Box 22.4 Effective HIV prevention strategies targeting injecting drug users**
>
> - Making sterile needles and syringes easily available
> - User-friendly, low-threshold drug treatment programmes, including oral methadone maintenance
> - Making access to HIV counselling and testing and post-exposure drug prophylaxis simple, for example, in syringe programmes facilities or hospital accident and emergency units
> - Sustained education through outreach programmes and peer education information, skills (for example, safer injecting), health services and social support
> - Facilitating access to health care, support and STD services for IDUs with HIV infection
> - Special programmes for high-risk subgroups (for example, sex workers, prison inmates, youths in detention)

Reducing HIV transmission through injecting relies on reducing the frequency of sharing of injecting equipment. Strategies that reduce injecting risk for HIV will have spin-off benefits for reducing other viral infections, for example hepatitis B and C. Social, political and legal controversies have hampered prevention strategies based on minimizing harm of injecting drug use to individuals and the community, because of concerns increasing the supply of clean injecting equipment would encourage injecting drug use. Evidence from observational evaluations shows this is unfounded. Research

has demonstrated that needle/syringe provision, that is providing sterile needles and syringes, is the most effective primary and secondary prevention strategy with drug users HIV uninfected and infected. Needle exchange has been successfully delivered in health and social services, through outreach workers and dispensing machines. It is associated with reduced HIV prevalence without increasing levels of drug use.

Improved access to bleach cleaning kits (for shared needles and syringes) and training in effective cleaning procedures may reduce transmission risk through needle sharing. However, it may be limited because of the quality of available products and the complex skills required. It is a poor substitute for access to clean needles, but better than no intervention at all.

Outreach and peer educators are the most effective way to reach drug users, and former and current injectors can be trained to perform these roles. Other interventions, specifically low-threshold easy-access drug treatment and oral methadone maintenance, can reduce overall levels of drug injecting. These interventions bring drug users into regular contact with service providers, where other interventions can be offered including STI and HIV testing, as well as routine outpatient HIV care for those with HIV. They also provide opportunities for adjunct social, educational and rehabilitation interventions to break the cycle of drug use.

## Conclusion

There are new and emerging opportunities for HIV prevention. However, the tried and tested methods of sustained condom use, reduction in number of sexual partners, and harm minimization in injecting drug use ensure that these established HIV prevention approaches will remain key to our response to HIV epidemics now and in the future.

## Further reading

AIDS Council of New South Wales, Australia produces highly effective communication strategies primarily targeting gay and other homosexually active men. (www.acon.org.au).

Center for AIDS Prevention Studies at the University of California at San Francisco. There is an extensive document library on effective HIV prevention strategies with diverse communities. (www.caps.ucsf.edu).

Terrence Higgins Trust is a key HIV/AIDS advocacy and service organisation with a wide range of essential HIV prevention information. (www.tht.org.uk).

United States Centers for Disease Control and Prevention (CDC). The website offers an extensive array of practical and policy information as well as detailed surveillance data. (www.cdc.gov/hiv).

# CHAPTER 23

# Patient and Community Perspective

*G. Brough[1] and N. Lubega[2]*

[1] Bloomsbury Clinic, Mortimer Market Centre, London, UK
[2] Patient Representative, London, UK

## Garry Brough

I have been HIV positive for over 20 years – I was infected in 1990, then found out I was HIV positive in 1991 at the age of 23, and went on to receive an AIDS diagnosis in 1995. I have experienced oral candida, Kaposi sarcoma (KS) (first cutaneous, then pulmonary), pneumocystis pneumonia (PCP), meningitis, septicaemia and a CD4 nadir of 10 cells/μL, but managed to stay alive until effective medication became available to deal with the virus. This was in no small part due to a winning combination of two consecutive doctors who were willing to have a two-way partnership with their patient, lots of support from friends and family, a positive attitude and outlook and the determination to do whatever it took to get through it all.

The prognosis for those diagnosed today is thankfully a very different story due to the huge advances in medication over the last 15 years. However, although HIV treatment can control the physical symptoms, the psychosocial issues that surround a positive HIV diagnosis remain, and understanding these is of critical importance to good patient care. HIV is an infectious disease and infected individuals worry about who to tell, how to tell, what reaction they will receive, will they be able to have a sexual partner or have children, will they face discrimination or be thought ill of. The stigma and fear that still accompany an HIV-positive diagnosis are real and involve sensitive issues, and until we reach a time when *everyone* is comfortable enough with HIV to consider it a 'manageable condition like diabetes' (to use an oft-quoted comparison), a model of care which is solely medical will always fall short. HIV continues to disproportionately affect people in the UK who are often marginalized or disempowered and the impact of this should neither be ignored nor underestimated. There is still an urgent need for education and support to those groups most affected as well as education for the general public and unfortunately within the NHS itself, where knowledge is variable, to say the least.

In recognition of the complexity of these issues, the role of patient advocacy and peer support are now considered an integral part of good patient care in many HIV services in the UK.

HIV has massively influenced the medical model of patient care. In the 1980s and early 1990s, HIV attracted an enormous amount of stigma and, due to the lack of effective treatment, there was greater focus on attempting to manage opportunistic infections and helping patients live (and die) as comfortably as possible than on treating HIV itself. This particularly difficult situation of seeing so many young people die, however, meant that services were adapted to meet the needs of patients. While this change was probably most visibly manifested in the way that AIDS wards were run, with the relaxation of the usual hospital rules (open visiting hours, made-to-order meals, nurses out of uniform and a general focus on the patient's comfort), it also created a unique opportunity for a different kind of doctor–patient relationship. First and foremost, the fact of having a designated clinician was a major advance from the earlier days of seeing whichever doctor happened to be available on a given day – when it wasn't unusual to see four different doctors over the course of a year's appointments. Continuity of care was recognized as an important factor in the patient's wellbeing, and this in turn led to a shift in the doctor–patient relationship, given that the physician not only got to know the specific circumstances and history of their patient, but that the patient was able to develop a stronger rapport with their doctor. There was more of a partnership than ever before, since in many instances the clinicians were as much in the dark about possible health issues as their (often highly informed) patients.

This shift from a 'doctor knows best' approach towards a more collaborative process made for a more relaxed, and in my experience, a far more trusting relationship than I would have previously believed possible. To have a belief that there were things that I could personally do to maintain my health and prolong my life was an essential element in my survival, and to have my HIV physician support and show an interest in the different approaches I tried was massively empowering.

When faced with doctors from specialities other than HIV, however, the contrast was often stark. I recall a heated debate with an oncologist who had recommended an aggressive experimental drug, since the chemotherapy was no longer managing the KS on my skin and in my lungs. I argued that there was no problem with the doxorubicin that I had been receiving, only that it needed to be put back to its original 3-weekly cycle instead of the 4-weekly cycle he had changed it to, but was told that this was nonsense, that he had no experience of just 1 week making a difference and that this could not affect the effectiveness of the treatment. My HIV clinician, however, knew perfectly well that I would refuse the new treatment and confirmed that I was entitled to choose to have the

*ABC of HIV and AIDS*, Sixth Edition. Edited by Michael W. Adler,
Simon G. Edwards, Robert F. Miller, Gulshan Sethi and Ian G. Williams.
© 2012 Blackwell Publishing Ltd. Published 2012 by Blackwell Publishing Ltd.

current therapy at the intervals that had previously been prescribed. I returned to 3-weekly cycles of doxorubicin and the KS stabilized again. I have no doubt that many doctors would have considered me a 'difficult' patient for insisting on this level of involvement in the decision-making process (I was never seen by that particular oncologist again!), but in the field of HIV at that time it was allowed and encouraged by HIV clinicians and nurses.

Although I am in no way proposing a switch from a 'doctor knows best' to a 'patient knows best' scenario, there is a great deal to be said for having the combined knowledge of doctor *and* patient when making decisions. The reason I emphasize this point is that with the arrival of cART, the power to dispense life-saving medication could easily lead HIV physicians back to a situation where 'consultations' are nothing of the sort, and we end up back in the days of 'take two of these and you'll feel much better' without any of the discussion of what a patient's needs might really be. In my day-to-day peer support work, patients often complain to me when they feel their doctors have not listened and responded appropriately to their problems and symptoms. Unfortunately, this usually happens after an eventual diagnosis is made, and the complaint often relates to the length of time they feel that their symptoms have been ignored or dismissed.

Frank and open doctor–patient dialogue is of paramount importance when it comes to prescribing cART, since ensuring an optimal first-line treatment regimen requires having all of the relevant information about a patient's general health, lifestyle and needs. Simply prescribing according to treatment guidelines and without a thorough knowledge of the patient will increase the risk of treatment failure, either because of adverse side effects, drug interactions or issues with adherence.

This whole process of involving the patient in the decision-making process is now informing the way the NHS works as a whole, and I believe that the example set by HIV services prepared the ground for the current shift towards a 'patient-led NHS'. Although this is now changing the way services will be delivered throughout the whole of the NHS, it would be a terrible shame to lose what has been gained through those bleak early years of the HIV epidemic at the basic level of the consultation. Those who worked with their consultants to achieve the best possible health outcomes, even in the face of impending death, have left a legacy of involvement in the process of healing which is essential to the doctor–patient relationship.

## Namatovu Lubega

This is the story of how I have been affected by my HIV diagnosis, my experiences and journey of living with HIV since 2005. HIV has been around me since the 1980s: I lost three sisters between 1993 and 2004. I have lost numerous other family members and in a lot of ways it is a personal tragedy. Although it has been a roller coaster, on a positive note, I have recovered well and had to accept and be comfortable with the fact that it will be a recovery in baby steps back to my old self. As a lot of people with HIV infection will know, HIV is as much a medical as an emotional, social and psychological condition.

My aim of sharing this story is to recognize the individuality of HIV testing and of living with HIV.

I will cover

- late diagnosis
- care and treatment outside of the HIV setting and its implications for HIV patients and their doctors
- HIV testing for children
- the social and psychological impact of HIV infection
- examples of good practice.

## Late diagnosis

Early diagnosis of HIV is the magical message for treatment and care, it is the preferred and ideal option. I would like to write this experience as the fairy tale whereby my infection was diagnosed early and I took advantage of the antiretroviral treatment available and had a successful and sustained immune recovery. However, that is not the case. I was aware of the facts about HIV, and had seen and supported a lot of people cope with the diagnosis. In my experience, all those I had come across had experienced HIV-related symptoms in one form or other, often many years before the actual diagnosis. This, I think, played a major factor in my late diagnosis in that I was completely asymptomatic up to my diagnosis. I did not have any history of illness and had a trouble-free pregnancy a few years before my diagnosis.

Worryingly, I even travelled to Africa having received live travel vaccines with what turned out to be a depleted immune system and still had no alarm bells.

I began feeling unwell in July 2004 with nothing outwardly related to HIV. A pain in my right hip was thought to be a muscle strain by the GP and some non-specific symptoms of feeling unwell. Emotionally I was slowly losing myself by the day. I was beginning to visit my GP with increasing frequency. I then acquired oral thrush in February 2005. This is when HIV infection came into the equation. I took the HIV test immediately and was found to be HIV positive. My doctors and I were shocked to find my CD4 count was only 10 cells/μL.

It is hard for me to work out whether I had HIV for a very long period of time or whether I contracted it in a few years and progressed quickly. I don't know at what point I could have been exposed. HIV is an individual infection, it affects people differently and the patterns are constantly changing. What I find difficult is constantly being asked by people 'Do you know how or when you acquired HIV?' This occurs more frequently in the medical setting than in the community. It often seems that these questions are to satisfy curiosity rather than enhance my care.

## Care and treatment outside of the HIV setting and its implications for HIV patients and their doctors

Late diagnosis, long-term side effects of HIV drugs and age mean that HIV patients will increasingly use services outside of the HIV settings. I have had my fair share of these experiences, and to date I have been treated in oncology, haematology, neurology, cardiology and associated services such as community nursing, speech therapy, cardiac rehabilitation and dietetics. I have been in hospital lots of times and have used A&E on numerous occasions. Up to 2011, I can confidently say that HIV treatment and care is a bubble where everything works: the patients and doctors work together in a partnership, the monitoring of patients is satisfactory, the communication and referrals are well processed and all supporting medical staff are aware of patient needs.

For infections that are associated with the diagnosis, close links with the HIV doctors have been developed over the years and this works well for HIV patients. However, this mainly applies to senior doctors. In my experience, staff who work in medical rotations such as junior doctors and registrars sometimes struggle to recognise that HIV patients need to be diagnosed and treated within the context of HIV, whatever the presenting problem. Communication with an HIV doctor can be really helpful to make sure an HIV-related diagnosis is not missed and that a treatment is not given that causes my HIV treatment to stop working.

I had an experience in hospital whereby a diagnosis wasn't taken in an HIV context. The gynaecologist on-call referred me to the outpatient clinic for which there was a nearly 2-month wait to be seen. My notes clearly said I had HIV infection and my HIV treatment centre was a few yards away from the hospital. In the waiting period I had an emergency for another illness and ended up on an HIV ward where the same medical illness turned out to be cytomegalovirus retinitis as diagnosed by the HIV clinicians. If my HIV clinic had been contacted when my gynaecological problem first occurred, then maybe I wouldn't be partially sighted in one eye. From then on I have given myself responsibility to make sure my HIV doctors are included in my care in any clinical setting. This is not always easy. It takes character and empowerment of patients and understanding of clinicians outside of HIV to agree to take the time to contact the HIV doctors.

General population illnesses are starting to take hold in the HIV population as we deal with the long-term side effects of drugs and age. In my experience this is where the main challenge lies. There is an increasing need to improve working relationships and treatment pathways for people with HIV presenting with illness outside of the HIV setting. At present the services are fragmented and systems independent. Traditionally clinicians in acute settings write to GPs to update them on any medical interventions with patients. However, HIV-positive patients are receiving ongoing care from two sources – their GP and their HIV clinic. I was recently treated in a non-HIV setting and found out that my GP was sent a letter summarizing the treatment I received but not my HIV doctor. There are two issues of concern here: first it is possible that my GP is not aware of my HIV status (this would be a breach of confidentiality), and second my HIV doctor doesn't have the information he needs to make the right decisions about my HIV treatment and ongoing monitoring. I have requested that letters be sent to him and nothing has happened. I do have a good relationship with my doctor and a basic understanding of treatment pathways and do report back to him as necessary. This is not ideal and shouldn't be happening. Not all patients can do this. Technology is available to enable coordinated decision-making among clinicians, whatever the speciality.

## HIV testing for children

I am a mother of two children. At the time of my diagnosis my daughter was 14 years and my son was 4 years old. They were both normal deliveries and breastfed up to 11 months. Both of them have no history of illness outside the normal childhood illnesses. I had no second thoughts about testing them, but when to do it was the challenge. I was very ill myself and since they did not have clinical symptoms I put it off until I was emotionally and physically ready. I tested my youngest child (age 7) first. This was during a summer holiday, and thankfully he was negative. My daughter was 17 years at the time and I didn't tell her about her brother or my diagnosis. A year later after a great deal of thought about her starting university and living an independent life (as well evidence from my doctor that children as old as 15 years were now presenting with HIV) I took the decision to sit down with my daughter and tell her about my status, her brother and the benefits of her taking the HIV test during the following summer holiday. This was against the advice of her dad who up to now doesn't know that she took the test or that we ever had this discussion. The emphasis was on mother-to-child transmission. She is negative and I am very happy with the decision to test my children.

## Social and psychological impact: examples of good practice

Living with HIV has a social and psychological impact on patients.

HIV has remained in certain groups of people and with it comes all the issues associated with marginalization.

- Sensitivity and respect are vital to HIV patients. They are normally well informed and questions like 'How did you get HIV?' are deemed offensive. Once a doctor in A&E told me 'if I was normal like him, he would discharge me without medication, but since I have HIV I need antibiotics'. I didn't need the antibiotics and didn't take them. Apart from being unacceptable language it was dangerous practice. Non-HIV doctors need to keep up with the changes of the epidemic and its impact on patient care.
- Testing for partners and children are discussed in the HIV and antenatal settings. Unless relevant to medical examinations, treatment or care they can appear judgemental and intrusive in non-HIV settings.
- HIV patients are likely to want to see their doctors or at least ensure there is adequate communication with them. In my experience this can be viewed as demanding by non-HIV doctors. I do think this is a reasonable request and I have experienced difficulties both in diagnosis and treatment when my HIV doctors are not involved.
- Confidentiality: this applies a lot to public waiting areas and wards. I had my HIV status disclosed to a friend visiting me in a non-HIV ward by a doctor giving me scan results. I have never discussed it with this person. I see them and pretend it didn't happen.

An ageing HIV-positive population means increasing care and treatment in non-HIV settings. Strategies and clinical practice to include HIV doctors in the care of patients is more urgent than ever. In my group of HIV-positive friends we call the HIV doctors *bakabaka* – the people in the know. The medical profession needs to be flexible about the treatment and care of patients with HIV.

# CHAPTER 24

# The Role of Patient Engagement

*C. Sandford*

Bloomsbury Clinic, Mortimer Market Centre, London, UK

**OVERVIEW**

- In the UK, there is a legal duty on all NHS trusts to involve and consult with patients
- Patient engagement can have a positive impact on physical and psychological health
- Patient involvement ranges from patient surveys, workshops, advocacy and peer support to formal representation in clinical management groups
- Well-informed patients are better able to take responsibility for their health and utilize more effectively the health services available
- Patients can play a role in the design of clinical services, which can have benefits for patients, staff and the wider NHS
- Special attention needs to be given to seek patient involvement from the wider patient group, specifically those with disabilities (hearing and/or visual impairment, learning difficulties and housebound), those who do not speak English as their first language and those at extremes of age

## Introduction

Patient engagement is now seen as a vital activity in the UK. It can have a positive impact on the physical health and psychological wellbeing of the patient in dealing effectively with both HIV diagnosis and ongoing care.

In turn, this will have a positive impact on their partners, friends, family, the wider community and improve the working relationship with their healthcare team. Their care becomes a collaborative process.

This chapter discusses the role of HIV patient engagement within the UK, but many of the issues raised are pertinent to care in any setting.

In 2010, the UK government published the White Paper 'Equity and Excellence: Liberating the NHS', which emphasized the involvement of patients in their care.

The key slogan 'no decision about me without me' reinforces the idea of patient choice and patient involvement. The aim is to create an environment whereby services are more responsive to patients needs and designed around them, rather than patients having to fit around services. This is supported by an increase in the amount of information made available to patients. In essence better informed patients are more likely to take an interest in their ongoing care.

In best practice, patient engagement means that patients work in partnership with clinicians, and take responsibility for adherence to medication and maintaining both physical health and psychological wellbeing.

Patient engagement can go further. People living with HIV – and those with other chronic conditions – become expert patients because of their regular contact with their clinic and healthcare teams. They can have a great deal of positive input into service planning, delivery and operation.

Indeed the law upholds this idea. Section 242 of the NHS Act 2006 places a legal duty on NHS Trusts and Strategic Health Authorities to involve and consult patients on a range of issues.

## How can services engage patients? (Box 24.1)

Patient engagement is initially the responsibility of the clinic. It begins with the healthcare team valuing the benefits of patient involvement and having a commitment to seeking their opinions and advice on service delivery.

This is further helped by the healthcare team taking the time to explain, to provide information and support at the time of diagnosis and throughout their patients' care – keeping them informed of new medical developments and offering counselling or psychosocial support as necessary.

Specific techniques for obtaining patient engagement are varied. One of the most frequently used methods is through collecting feedback via surveys, questionnaires, evaluation forms and focus groups. These can make the patient feel valued, a key part of the team and a useful source of feedback on service provision.

Patient involvement can be invaluable where the remit is to review or design a patient pathway within a service. However wonderful the department might look to a health employee, some newly diagnosed HIV-positive patients may be too scared to cross the threshold into the HIV clinic or find navigating aspects of the service very daunting and stigmatizing.

*ABC of HIV and AIDS*, Sixth Edition. Edited by Michael W. Adler,
Simon G. Edwards, Robert F. Miller, Gulshan Sethi and Ian G. Williams.
© 2012 Blackwell Publishing Ltd. Published 2012 by Blackwell Publishing Ltd.

Journey mapping using patient involvement can help identify how the service really appears to patients and simple measures can be put in place that can make a big difference to the patient experience.

Other forms of engagement which can be encouraged by the clinic are based on *peer support*. These can include patient networks, forums, social events, interactive websites, workshops, newly diagnosed courses and the introduction of salaried patient representatives.

All these activities engage patients in their care, emphasize what the patient can do to help themselves and provide peer support, advice and advocacy on a range of issue outside the medical remit but of great importance to patients.

## What are the advantages for patients and care providers?

### Patients

Diagnosis with HIV can be accompanied by suicidal thoughts, loss of self-esteem, confidence and trust. It can lead to self-stigmatization, anxiety and fear for the future, which in turn can lead to withdrawal and social isolation.

Engagement of a patient at the earliest opportunity and making sure they have the correct information and support can help stop these negative feelings developing into more serious concerns.

The advantages to the patient can be summarized as

* empowerment through information
* reduction in anxiety and fear
* increased confidence, self-awareness and self-esteem
* increased trust in healthcare professionals
* greater understanding of the importance of psychological well-being
* greater understanding of the importance of physical health and lifestyle choices
* patients can gain a greater understanding of the service and how to use it effectively.

## Care providers

If the patient is engaged in their care, the healthcare professionals have an opportunity for continuous improvement and redesign of services through feedback and evaluation to provide the best care model for their patients.

The advantages of patient engagement for the clinician can be summarized as

* improved understanding of patients' health concerns
* improved understanding of the impact of diagnosis
* greater awareness of coping skills
* expert patient feedback on services
* informs continuous improvement and redesign of services
* informs criteria, standards and guideline setting
* involvement can help to shape future services and the clinic space to promote a healthy environment for all patients.

## Peer support

Peer support, advice, advocacy and means of engagement can be provided by statutory and non-statutory organizations. The advantages of peer support in a clinical setting include continuity of care and involvement in providing continuous and knowledgeable feedback on service provision.

### Patient representatives

It is well recognized that doctor–patient consultations are time limited and are not able to cover all the issues that are important to the patient. In addition, a patient may not feel empowered or comfortable raising certain personal or sensitive information with their clinician.

Patient representatives offer an additional opportunity where important HIV-related issues such as safer sex, disclosure, fears of stigma and discrimination can be raised. They also provide another mechanism for patient feedback on the quality of the service.

Patient clinics can be staffed by salaried patient representatives (there are a number of HIV clinics in the UK which do this). There are many others who volunteer their services in clinics throughout the country.

Patient representatives offer peer support, advice, advocacy and means of engagement.

Services can be delivered through a regular drop in and appointment service.

Positive outcomes of peer support include

* offering a patient's perspective to living with the virus
* offering empathy not sympathy
* addressing psychosocial issues not covered in medical consultations
* offering practical and emotional support through statutory and non-statutory organizations
* addressing patients anxieties about access and treatment
* addressing patients' low self-esteem and confidence – motivation, empowering and engaging
* addressing patients' anxieties about being able to live a normal life.

Patient representatives may also be involved in teaching, committees – local and national – and representing patients at management level.

## Representation at management meetings

Management meetings are often places where key changes to services are discussed. Patient representation at these meetings affords an opportunity to ensure that service changes are developed in consultation with patients. They can ensure that issues pertinent to patients are put on the agenda such as opening hours, specific services and care pathways.

## Workshops

Workshops are held by a large number of voluntary organizations, including the Terrence Higgins Trust, Body & Soul and Positively UK. They are also offered within some HIV services via local patient network e.g., the Bloomsbury Patient Network at the Mortimer Market Centre, London.

Workshops offer engagement and empowerment through information and learning, dealing with issues not traditionally covered in the medical model but of great importance to patients – for instance, disclosure, building self-esteem, positive thinking, and love, sex and relationships.

By engaging in workshops and meeting other people living with the virus a patient realizes they are not alone.

Other positive outcomes include

- increased knowledge about living positively
- less fear and anxiety
- increased disclosure
- a social and support network leading to less isolation
- feeling of being more in control
- increasing self-awareness and addressing self-stigmatization
- a feeling of being better to engage with life.

## Forums

Forums provide a basis for the dissemination of information, a platform for discussion and debate, providing feedback to providers, political organizations and professional bodies.

Forums happen both online–www.myhiv.org.uk or www.forum-link.org – or are held by organizations such as NAM. They often focus on issues that are deemed to be of high importance to patients and are generally complementary to information provided elsewhere, e.g. *Engagement with Primary Care, Medical Updates, The Impact of NHS Reforms.*

Forums not only inform the patient but also have an impact on professional organizations and national policy at all levels. For example, organizations that have attended events where I am based (the Mortimer Market Centre) include: Royal College of General Practitioners, British Medical Association, Metropolitan Police, British Dental Association, Medical Foundation for AIDS & Sexual Health (MedFASH), British HIV Association, London Specialist Commissioning Group and the All Party Parliamentary Group on HIV.

## Newly diagnosed courses

Courses for the newly diagnosed are available from some HIV services and a variety of voluntary organizations.

These courses provide information, support and advice at a crucial moment in people's lives and allow participants to feel they are not alone. They are invaluable in helping patients come to terms with their diagnosis and provide a forum to discuss key issues with trained facilitators. Other aims of these courses are

- encouraging a feeling of safety and belonging
- improving knowledge and understanding
- correcting misconceptions, urban myths, misinformation and negative language
- exploring past and present fears and anxieties
- realizing that every problem is not attributable to HIV
- exploring irrational fears vs rational thought
- greater acceptance of diagnosis
- improved psychological and physical wellbeing
- self-management and life skills
- confidence in disclosing status.

## Social events

Patients groups and patient representatives all over the country organize social events that provide a means to meet and discuss issues of the day – often with a guest speaker – to socialize, relax and have some fun. In London such social events are organized by Str8talk, Positively UK, Gay Men's Group, THT, Positive East and Bloomsbury Patients Network at the Mortimer Market Centre.

## Conclusions

Patient engagement can have a major impact on people's physical health and psychological wellbeing.

- It encourages the patient to take an active role in a collaborative process rather than be a passive victim.
- It encourages the patient to take responsibility for themselves, for adherence and for those around them
- In turn this engagement will have a positive impact on their partners, friends, family, the wider community, their healthcare team and service providers
- An engaged, well-informed patient will have a greater sense of being in control, will not self-stigmatize or consider themselves a victim and will live a more positive and fulfilling life.

# Index

Numbers in *italics* refer to figures; numbers in **bold** refer to tables.

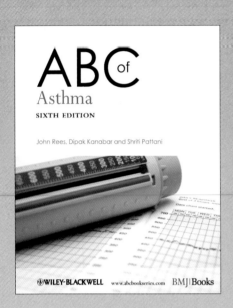

# ABC of Asthma

## 6TH EDITION

### John Rees, Dipak Kanabar & Shriti Pattani
Guy's Hospital, London; Guy's Hospital, London; North West London Hospitals NHS Trust

- This new edition has been thoroughly revised with reference to the latest British Thoracic Society guidelines on the management of asthma in children and adults

- Provides a concise, up-to-date overview of all aspects of asthma and includes two new chapters focussing on GP practice issues including clinical management and organisation of asthma care

- Covers the advances in practice and methods, with a new emphasis on delivery systems, self-dose assessment and delivery of care with different pharmacological approaches

- Ideal for GPs, junior doctors and medical students, nurses, and anyone dealing with the treatment of asthma in children and adults

APRIL 2010 | 9781405185967 | 104 PAGES | £26.99/US$39.95/€34.90/AU$54.95

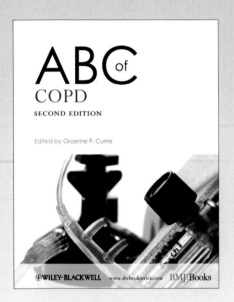

# ABC of COPD

## 2ND EDITION

### Edited by Graeme P. Currie
Aberdeen Royal Infirmary

- Chronic Obstructive Pulmonary Disease (COPD) is a progressive, irreversible lung disease and one of the most common medical conditions necessitating admission to hospital and ongoing management within primary care

- Provides a practical and relevant account of COPD, together with improved guidance on effective diagnosis, management and treatment of this common and progressive disorder

- Thoroughly updated and includes new chapters on the correct use of inhalers, oxygen, issues in primary care, and palliative care and end of life issues commonly faced by those suffering from COPD

- Includes a new section of case histories to illustrate how chapter contents can be practically applied

- An authoritative and practical guide for general practitioners, practice nurses, nurses sitting the CODP diploma, medical students, paramedical staff, junior doctors and health professionals working in primary care

DECEMBER 2010 | 9781444333886 | 88 PAGES | £22.99/US$35.95/€29.90/AU$47.95